The Cytotoxics Handbook

Edited for
The Cytotoxics Services Working Group by

Michael Allwood

BPharm, PhD, MRPS, Director of Pharmacy Research and
Development, Medicines Research Unit, Southern Derbyshire
Health Authority, Derby

and

Patricia Wright

BPharm, MPhil, MRPS, Principal Pharmacist,
The Royal London Hospital (Whitechapel), London

RADCLIFFE MEDICAL PRESS
OXFORD

© 1990 Radcliffe Medical Press Ltd
15 Kings Meadow, Ferry Hinksey Road, Oxford OX2 0DP

British Library Cataloguing in Publication Data

The Cytotoxics Handbook
  1. Man. Effects of drugs. Cytotoxics
  I. Allwood, M.C. (Michael Charles) 1943- II. Wright, Patricia
  615.7

ISBN 1 870905 61 X

Printed in Great Britain at the Alden Press, Oxford

Contents

PART TWO

Drug Monographs: Compendium of Intravenous Drugs in Cancer Chemotherapy

Investigational Drugs

The past 20 to 25 years have witnessed impressive changes in the drug treatment of cancer.

A better understanding of the nature of neoplastic disease has led to the development of cancer chemotherapeutic drugs, encompassing a wide spectrum of chemical compounds, which kill or impair susceptible tumour cells by blocking a drug-sensitive biochemical or metabolic pathway. The ability to use a number of agents in combination has improved clinical outcome in a variety of conditions and increasingly complex regimens continue to be developed.

However, cytotoxic therapy has its limitations: poor selectivity between neoplastic and normal cells, especially in the bone marrow and reproductive organs, can produce severe side-effects; many of the agents are carcinogens and mutagens and have been implicated in causing secondary neoplasms in patients being treated for cancer and most agents cause local damage to skin and mucous membranes due to their irritant, vesicant or allergenic action.

The obvious toxicity of these drugs has led to concern over their possible toxicity to healthcare workers who prepare and administer the drugs and care for the patients during treatment. In response to a number of reports indicating skin absorption and droplet inhalation of cytotoxics prepared in uncontrolled environments, guidelines for the safe handling of antineoplastic drugs have been drawn up by a number of countries. All make the same basic recommendations: controlled handling procedures; a high level of staff training and, where practicable, centralized reconstitution of IV cytotoxics in a pharmacy department with suitable controlled working areas.
In the UK, The Control of Substances Hazardous to Health Regulations (1988) require employers, by law, to prevent or control exposure of employees (or of visitors to their premises) to any substances potentially or actually hazardous to health. Hence, the increasing need for cytotoxics to be handled in a controlled environment by informed staff.

The development of centralized pharmacy cytotoxic services over the last 10 years has occurred in a non-uniform manner depending on local requirements, the availability of funding and the existing service commitments. Where services have been established, much time has been spent researching the literature for information on drug stability, designing documentation, establishing training programmes and ensuring that facilities comply with Health and Safety requirements. That services have been established is commendable considering the general lack of information on the safe handling and stability of IV cytotoxics and the divergent and conflicting views of much published work.

In response to the obvious need for more practical information on the procedures involved in setting up and running such units, a group comprising pharmacists and technicians in the UK met for informal, 'round table' discussions in 1987. All members had a substantial interest and expertise in cytotoxic drugs and the development of pharmacy-based hospital cytotoxic services and represented hospital pharmacy, academic interests and the pharmaceutical industry. Early in the discussions, it was agreed that the Cytotoxic Services Working Group would produce a manual on how to set up and operate pharmacy-based cytotoxic services with specific detail on equipment, facilities, Health and Safety, documentation and training; and a compendium of cytotoxic drugs detailing their pharmaceutical properties, reconstitution details and stability in secondary packaging systems based on an informed review of the literature. A first edition was printed in late 1988.

This second edition has been extensively updated to reflect developments in the field of cytotoxic chemotherapy over the last three years. The manual and compendium are now combined into a single handbook designed primarily for use by pharmacists wishing to establish or update centralized cytotoxic services but will also be of use to other healthcare workers in this speciality.

Part one is divided into 10 chapters, each giving detailed information on a specific topic related to cytotoxic services. The information given is representative of the current 'state of the art' cytotoxic reconstitution services and reflects international recommendations and the contributors' own experience.

Part two is a compendium of monographs on injectable cytotoxic drugs. These monographs have been prepared for specific use by those hospital pharmacists and experienced pharmacy technicians who have responsibility for the provision of reconstituted and ready-to-administer cytotoxic drugs. Information on stability refers to preparation in controlled environments, where the sterility of the final product can be assured. The object of each monograph is to provide the basic information relevant to the preparation; stability on storage in the primary container; stability in secondary packaging systems; administration and disposal of the drugs. Use of the monographs should obviate the need for extensive literature searching and interpretation of data. The author of each monograph is named and can be consulted on specific queries.

Interferon, interleukins and granulocyte-stimulating factors are not included in the handbook because they do not have a direct cytotoxic action and can be handled safely.

Investigational agents will be kept under constant review and new drugs will be included in future editions to the handbook. For information on these agents, readers are referred to the National Cancer Institute book of Investigational Drugs (available from The Pharmaceutical Resources Branch, NCI, Executive Plaza North, Suite 818, Bethesda, Maryland, 20892, USA) and specialist oncology centres.

Michael C. Allwood
Director of Pharmacy Research & Development
Medicines Research Unit
Derby Royal Infirmary
Derby

Susan E. Ayers
Pharmacist
Oncology & Bone Marrow Transplant Services
Pharmacy Department
St. James University Hospital
Leeds

Rosamund M. Baird
Consultant in Pharmaceutical Microbiology
Summerlands House
Summerlands
Yeovil

Nigel Ballentine
Principal Pharmacist, Clinical Services
Pharmacy Department
Birmingham Children's Hospital
Birmingham

Kay A. Buttars
Chief Technician
Pharmacy Department
Addenbrookes Hospital
Cambridge

Christine L. Chard
Oncology Business Manager
Degussa Pharmaceuticals Ltd
168, Cowley Road
Cambridge

Patrick F. D'Arcy
Research Adviser in Pharmacy
East Anglia Regional Health Authority, Cambridge &
    Visiting Professor University of London
Cambridge

Karen S. Davis
Intravenous Therapy Division
Baxter Healthcare Ltd
Compton
Newbury
Berks

Monica Francomb
Staff Pharmacist, Clinical Services
Royal Liverpool Hospital
Liverpool

Sarah A. Giles
Senior Medical Information Officer
Lederle Laboratories Ltd
Gosport
Hants

Ian J. Goss
Director of Operational Services
Pharmacy Department
Leeds General Infirmary
Leeds

Nigel M. Goulding
Principal Pharmacist
Pharmacy Department
Charing Cross Hospital
London

Pauline E. Heath
Commercial Development Manager
Bristol-Myers Co Ltd
Hounslow
Middlesex

A. Paul Launchbury
Technical Director
Farmitalia Carlo Erba Ltd
St. Albans
Herts

M. Gerard Lee
Regional Quality Controller
Pharmacy Department
Mersey Regional Health Authority
Liverpool

Tony C. Moore
Principal Pharmacist, Technical Services
Pharmacy Department
Royal Hallamshire Hospital
Sheffield

Richard J. Needle
Pharmacy Technical Support Manager
Pharmacy Support Unit
Colchester General Hospital
Colchester

Jonathan M. Oakes
Principal Pharmacist
Pharmacy Department
Countess of Chester Hospital
Chester

Nutan Patel
Chief Pharmacy Technician
Pharmacy Department
The Royal Marsden Hospital
London

Tim Root
Group Pharmacist
Pharmacy Department
The Royal Marsden Hospital
London

Graham J. Sewell
Principal Pharmacist & Senior Lecturer in
    Biomedical Sciences
Department of Pharmacy
Royal Devon & Exeter Hospital
Exeter

Robert J.S. Shaw
Regional Quality Controller
East Anglian Regional Pharmaceutical Services
Norfolk & Norwich Hospital
Norwich

Andrew P. Stanley
District Oncology Pharmacist
St. Chads Unit
Dudley Road Hospital
Birmingham

Helen R. Streeter
Pharmacist, Bone Marrow Transplant Services
Pharmacy Department
University Hospital of Wales
Cardiff

John V. Wilson
Senior Pharmacist, Research
Pharmacy Department
General Hospital
Nottingham

M. Jayne Wood
Senior Pharmacist, Research
Pharmacy Department
Queen Elizabeth Hospital
Birmingham

M. Patricia Wright
Principal Pharmacist
Pharmacy Department
The Royal London Hospital (Whitechapel)
London

CHAPTER 1

Setting up a Cytotoxic Reconstitution Service

Before proceeding, it is advisable to ask the following questions and collect relevant data.

1. IS THERE A NEED FOR SUCH A SERVICE?

1 Range of Service and Projected Workload

It will be necessary to establish:

The number and type of individual cytotoxic doses administered per annum and whether new types of therapy (eg continuous domiciliary) are likely to change workload patterns:

Who prescribes cytotoxic chemotherapy; where and when is it administered and by whom (eg are certificated nurses available to administer parenteral chemotherapy);

Is the workload continuous or does it fluctuate; at what time of day/week are particular regimens commenced;

Is bolus injection (manual or via syringe pump) or intravenous infusion the preferred method of administration?

2 Health and Safety Considerations

Where is cytotoxic reconstitution currently being carried out and by whom? Are these arrangements satisfactory and appropriate from a patient safety and operator protection point of view?

3 Cost

What is the current capital and revenue expenditure on cytotoxic chemotherapy (drugs, equipment, facilities and staff)?

Are significant amounts of medical and nursing time, that would better be utilized providing direct patient care, being devoted to the preparation of cytotoxic chemotherapy?

Will centralization of cytotoxic reconstitution produce economies of scale and reduce revenue expenditure?

4 Consultation

All interested parties (medical, nursing, administrative and pharmaceutical) should be approached for information and opinions. The choice of a formal or informal approach will depend on local circumstances and relationships.

5 Commitments and Resources

The present level of commitments and resources should
be examined before proceeding further. A centralized
reconstitution service is a major development and will require
either additional resources, or the redeployment of existing
resources. An awareness of local, district and regional strategic
plans is vital at this stage to ensure that an appropriate balance
of commitments to resources is achieved.

6 Collecting and Testing Data

A pilot scheme is an effective mechanism for collecting data,
canvassing opinions and testing logistics and procedures. Such
a scheme should have clear objectives, a fixed timescale and an
agreed endpoint when the results can be evaluated without
prejudice. A decision to proceed or not can then be made,
based on actual local experience.

Before starting a pilot study a multidisciplinary working party
should be established with a nominated co-ordinator.

---

2. SETTING UP A CYTOTOXICS WORKING PARTY

1 Membership

Membership of the working party should include:

Clinicians	Oncologists Haematologists Radiologists Radiotherapists
Nurses	Nurse managers Tutors Specialists Community
Pharmacy staff	Pharmacists (including District Pharmacist to ensure consistency across district) Technicians
Management	Unit general manager or representative
Occupational health	Senior representative

2 Objectives

▼ To establish and co-ordinate a pilot study in accordance with
previously agreed aims and objectives.
▼ To assess the capital and revenue implications of the service
and allocate resources as appropriate.
▼ To monitor the performance of the service.

It is desirable that a smaller working party should continue to
meet in the longer term to formulate policy and provide advice
on relevant issues.

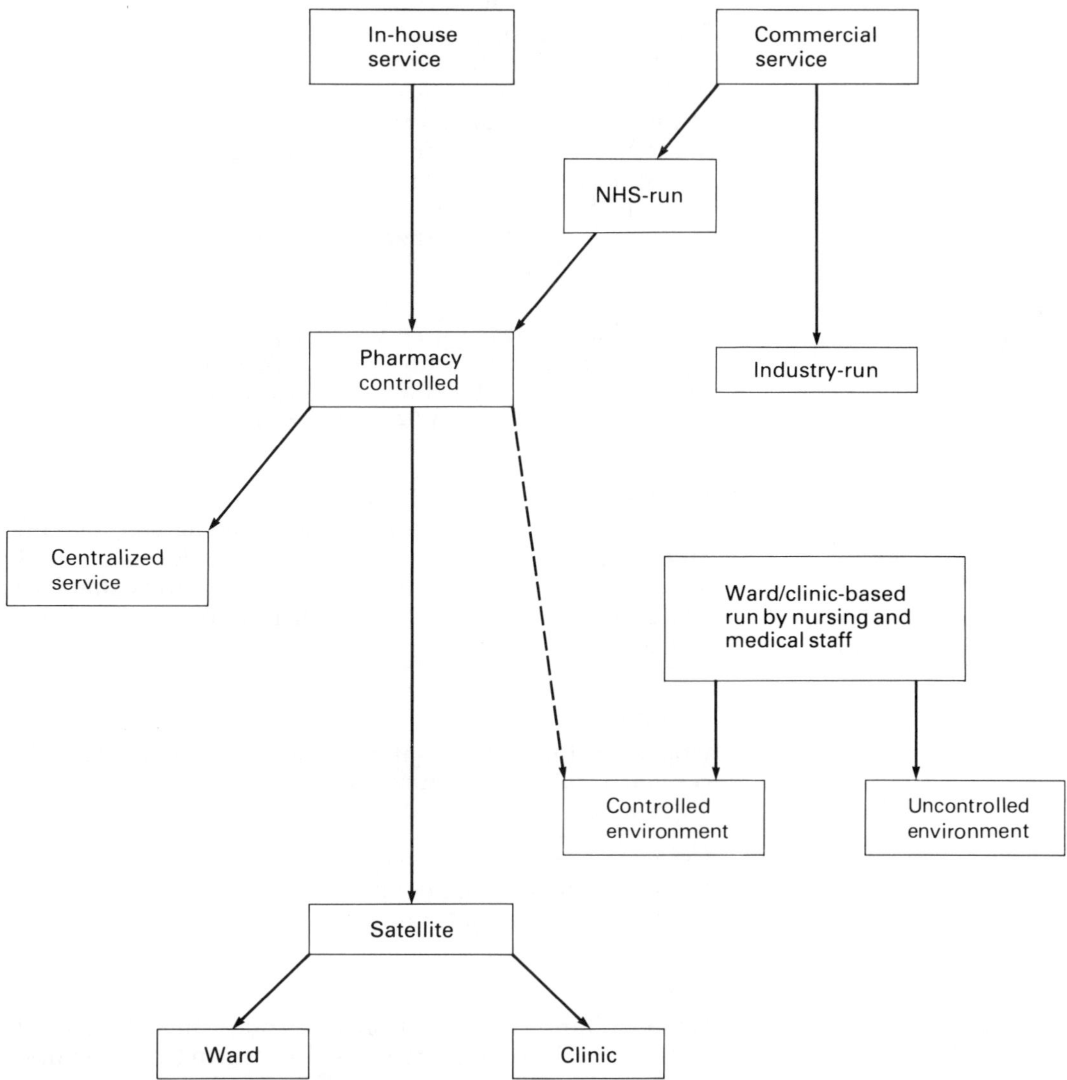

Figure 1.1: *Flow chart summarizing service selection criteria*

3. WHAT TYPE OF SERVICE IS REQUIRED?

An option appraisal is useful in determining the type of service required. Areas for consideration are outlined in Figure 1.1.

1 Service Selection Criteria

Workload

The volume of work, measured as individual patient doses per annum, and annual expenditure on cytotoxic chemotherapy are key considerations.

Range and presentation of doses

The range and pattern of cytotoxic prescribing needs to be determined. The key areas to consider are:
▼ the range of cytotoxics used;
▼ the stability in solution of the drugs used;
▼ methods of administration (eg bolus injections, infusions and continuous infusions);
▼ are treatment regimens established?
▼ is there any standardization of doses?

Level of service

Determine the level of service Pharmacy can provide. Will this give a total service in normal working hours? If not, can prescribing habits be changed to make such a service possible?
   Alternatively, does a 24 hour service need to be established?

Quality assurance and sterility assurance

Quality assurance procedures should be agreed, documented and adhered to. In order to achieve high levels of sterility assurance, procedures should include rigorous standards for equipment maintenance, operator training and environmental monitoring.

Facilities

Utilize existing facilities if available. If these are not available, convert facilities and purchase appropriate equipment.

Health and safety needs

Local and national guidelines must be adhered to
(*see* Chapter 6, Health and Safety).

Funding

Have resources been identified? If not, can potential savings on drug expenditure and medical and nursing time be utilized?
   What other developments are underway or being planned and what is the order of priority?

Personnel

Are there staff available and what is their level of expertise? Are funds available for recruitment and training?

Logistics

Points for consideration:

▼ the physical geography of the site/sites;
▼ is more than one site being serviced?
▼ location of in-patients and out-patients within the same site in relation to Pharmacy;
▼ communication and transport systems;
▼ consultants' prescribing habits.

Clinical commitment

The level of clinical involvement by Pharmacy can be enhanced by providing a service. This level of involvement with patient care should not detract from the efficiency of the service and will depend on the attitudes of local personnel and their managers.

4. DECIDING ON THE LEVEL OF SERVICE

Some of the advantages and disadvantages of each type of service are shown in Table 1.1.

Table 1.1: *Advantages and disadvantages of possible service options*

Service	Advantages	Disadvantages
Pharmacy controlled centralized unit	Existing facilities.	Potential large capital cost if using cleanroom technology.
	High sterility/stability assurance.	Extended lines of communication between Pharmacy/nurse/doctor.
	Cost/efficiency savings on a high workload.	Problems of distribution to clinical areas and off-site locations.
	Planned workload.	Slower reaction/lead times.
	Suitably trained, skilled staff.	Out of hours service may not be provided.
	High level of operator/product protection.	Potential long-term Pharmacy staff exposure.
	Easier supervision.	High level of long-term Pharmacy commitment.
	Standardization of presentation of doses.	Loss of expertise at ward level.
	Comprehensive documentation.	
Pharmacy controlled satellite unit	Workload centralized in designated hospital areas.	Deployment of staff away from Pharmacy, with the potential for increased staff requirements and labour costs.
	Short lines of communication.	Increased stock holdings.
	Reduced distribution problems.	Potential for greater wastage.
	Increased inter-professional contact.	Fragmentation of pharmacy service.

Table 1.1: *continued*

Service	Advantages	Disadvantages
	Ability to respond more quickly to requests.	Negotiating space within another department.
	Cost/efficiency savings on high workload.	May also be required to supply oral medication and adjuvant therapy.
	High sterility/stability assurance.	Potential long-term Pharmacy staff exposure.
	Easier to provide an extended hours service.	
	Potential for access by non-Pharmacy staff out of hours (working to strict Pharmacy procedures).	
	High level of operator/product protection.	
Ward/clinic based in an uncontrolled environment (nurse/ doctor operated)	Status quo.	Health and Safety aspects/ operator protection. No product protection. High level of wastage. High stock holdings. Limited Pharmacy control. No record of preparation process; therefore no recall traceability. Possibility of untrained staff preparing doses.
Ward/clinic based in a controlled environment (nurse/ doctor operated)	Reduced Pharmacy labour costs. Rapid response, 24-hour service. Short lines of communication. No distribution or delivery problems.	High nursing and medical staff turnover, leading to increased training requirements. Less time for direct patient care. Decreased assurance of sterility/stability. Higher level of wastage. Limited Pharmacy control. No record of preparation process; therefore no recall traceability.

Table 1.1: *continued*

Service	Advantages	Disadvantages
		Increased stock holdings.
		Difficult to maintain high standard of quality assurance.
		Pharmacy activity undertaken by non-Pharmacy staff.
		Management responsibilities and levels of control poorly defined.
		Formal accrediting/validation system would be required, which would lead to increased quality assurance costs.
Commercial service (industry/ NHS[1] based)	No additional capital or staff costs (full off-site service).	Potential for increased revenue expenditure.
	Provision of a full range of drugs in a ready-to-use form.	Some products prepared under a manufacturer's 'specials' licence.
	Health and safety aspects of local reconstitution eliminated.	Communication and supply logistics (if service off-site).
	Standardization of presentation of doses.	Further distribution of drugs from a central delivery point to the ward/clinic.
	Planned workload.	
	Comprehensive documentation.	
	Minimal stock holdings.	
	Reduced wastage.	
	High sterility/stability assurance.	

[1]If NHS-based, then see Pharmacy controlled centralized system, with the addition that such a service has the potential for revenue generation for the department.

Facilities

INTRODUCTION

The selection of equipment and working environment is dependent on a number of factors:

▼ expected workload
▼ existing facilities and commitments
▼ resources available (capital/revenue, personnel, accommodation)

The following flow chart (Figure 2.1) identifies options to be considered in the decision-making process.

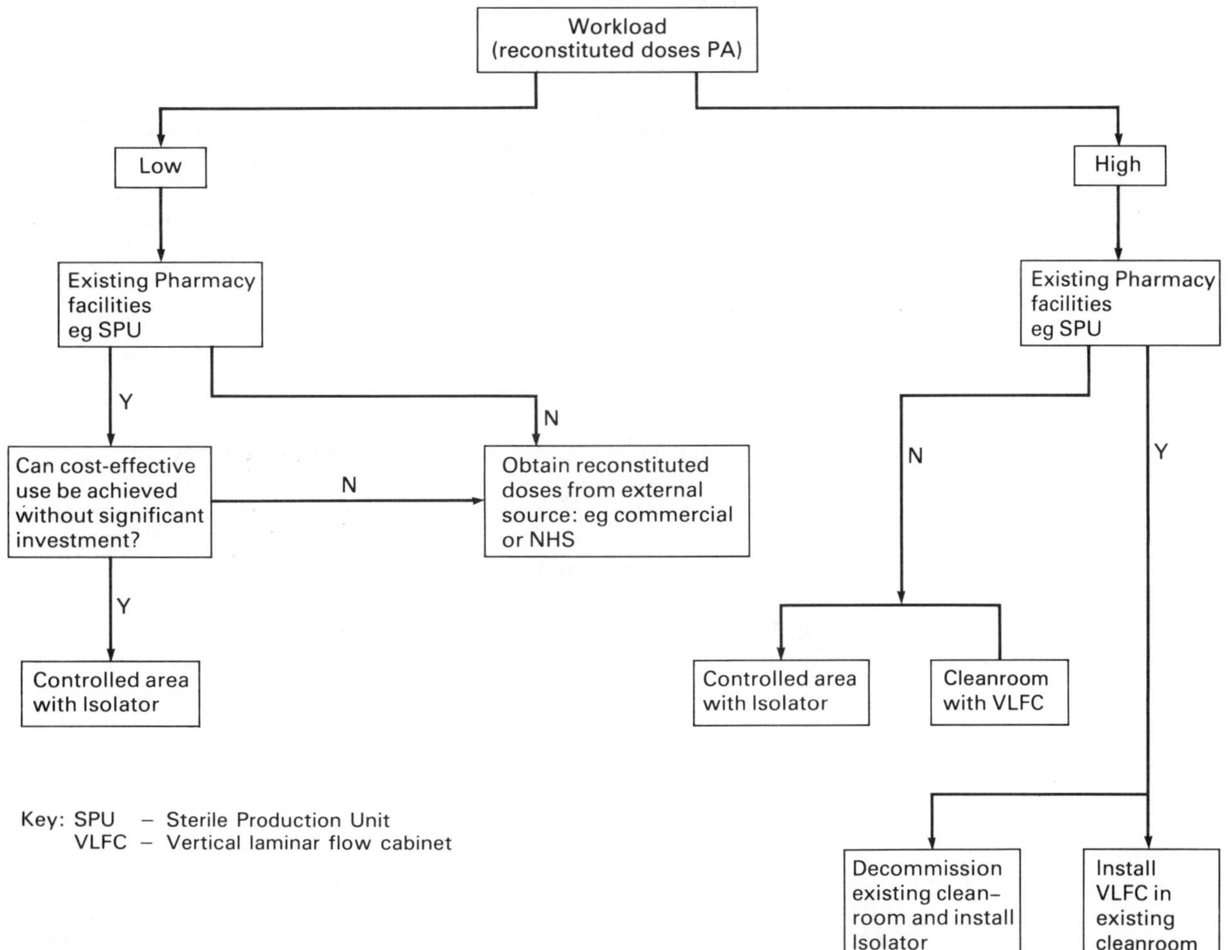

Figure 2.1: *Flow chart of options to be considered when selecting equipment and working environment*

VERTICAL LAMINAR FLOW CABINETS AND ISOLATORS

The risks associated with the handling and administration of cytotoxic drugs have resulted in the widespread use of safety cabinets for the preparation and dispensing of these products. Such cabinets must achieve a balance between operator and product protection in order to provide adequate levels of safety for both the patient and the staff preparing and administering the drug. Vertical laminar flow cabinets (VLFC) with similar operating characteristics to Class II microbiological safety cabinets have been used, but the limitations of these cabinets have led to an increased use of isolators (totally enclosed glove boxes). These have an advantage over cleanrooms in that they do not require an expensive air handling plant nor do they need costly and time-consuming gowning procedures.

1 Vertical Laminar Flow Cabinets

Standards

There are no nationally agreed standards in the U.K. for vertical laminar flow drug safety cabinets. The British Standard for Microbiological Safety Cabinets, BS 5726,[1] makes reference to vertical laminar flow protection cabinets, but this Standard is not readily applicable to hazardous drugs because:

▼ bacteria have a defined mass or bulk and are of known particle size, whereas cytotoxic contaminants will be of variable size and may be solid, liquid or gaseous
▼ for the materials handled in microbiological safety cabinets, operator protection is more critical than product protection

The Australian Standard, AS 2567, 1982[2] has been written to apply only to cytotoxic cabinets. Some of the features of this Standard are:

▼ all potentially contaminated zones are under negative pressure
▼ all filter seals which may come into contact with potentially hazardous material are under negative pressure with respect to the uncontaminated zones
▼ stainless steel construction
▼ incorporation of carbon exhaust filter.

Operating principles

A vertical downflow of laminar-flow air, filtered through a HEPA filter (99.997% efficiency), passes over the work surface. The air then passes through vents at the front and back of the cabinet, through another HEPA filter and is recirculated. Approximately 30% of the recirculated air is exhausted from the cabinet and, to compensate for this, air is drawn in through the front opening. This creates a negative pressure within the cabinet. The balance between the cabinet downflow and the air drawn in at the front of the cabinet produces an air curtain, which is the basis of the operator and product protection properties of the cabinet. The air exhausted from the cabinet may be recirculated into the room or ducted to the outside.

Cabinet details

Cytomat (Medical Air Technology Ltd)

Cabinet dimensions (w × d × h (mm)) 1200 × 695 × 2135

Tray area (w × d (mm)) 1075 × 450

Filters The Cytomat is available in two formats. The fixed format has a downflow HEPA filter, 1100 mm × 500 mm × 150 mm and an exhaust HEPA filter, 1000 mm × 450 mm × 300 mm. The movable format has an additional in-line exhaust HEPA filter, 825 mm × 375 mm × 75 mm. Filters are sealed on both the upstream and downstream faces.

Design characteristics The manufacturer states that this machine is built to AS 2567,[2] but it does not fully comply as the working chamber tank is not entirely of stainless steel construction. The air flow through the cabinet is generated by a fan in the terminal exhaust duct; therefore the cabinet and exhaust system will be under negative pressure. The ducting is fitted with anti-blowback flaps. The filter case forms the walls of the air ducts; therefore air cannot bypass the filter. The exhaust duct can be fitted with either a carbon or an HEPA exhaust filter.

Figure 2.2 shows the airflow pattern for the total dumping (exhaust) and recirculating versions of this cabinet.

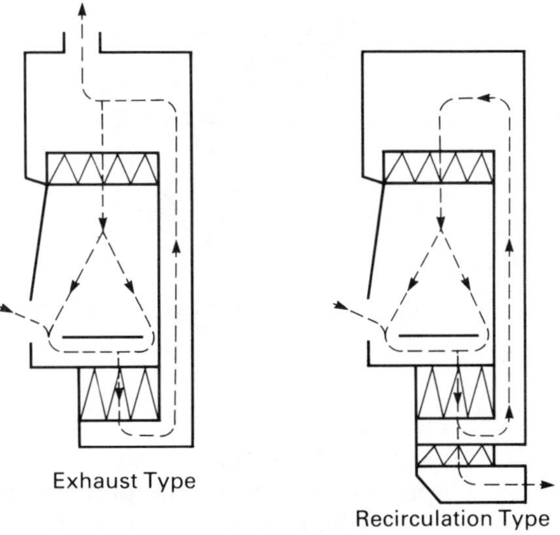

Figure 2.2: *M.A.T. Cytomat airflow diagram*

Cytogard (Gelman Hawkseley Ltd)

Cabinet dimensions (h × w × d (mm)) w × d × h
model CG 900 – 2310 × 1180 × 768 1180 × 768 × 2310
model CG 120 – 2310 × 1340 × 770 1340 × 770 × 2310
model CH 180 – 2310 × 1950 × 770 1950 × 770 × 2310

Tray area (CG 900) (w × d (mm)) 875 × 590

Filters Filters are Gelman microseal 7531 series (dimensions not stated). One downflow HEPA filter and one exhaust HEPA filter are fitted, plus an activated carbon bed in the exhaust. The exhaust filter is sealed on the upstream face.

Design characteristics This cabinet complies with AS 2567.[2] The cabinets are bulkier and taller than the Cytomat. They have no normal provision for exhaust ducting, but this can be done. Manometers are optional and do not allow measurement downstream of the main filter. Some bypassing of the upper (product protection) filter has been reported.

Figure 2.3 shows the airflow pattern for this type of cabinet.

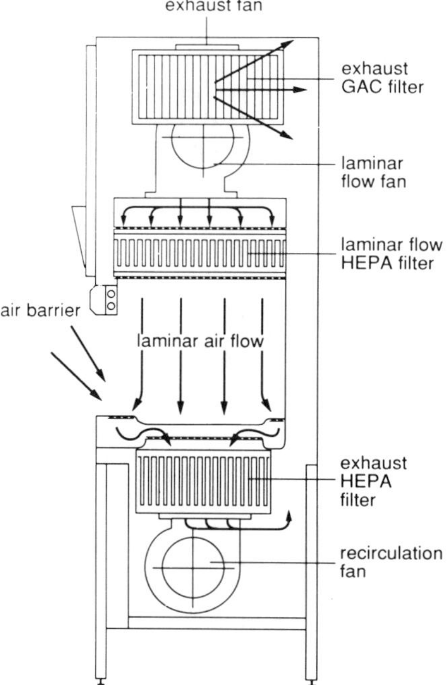

Figure 2.3: *Gelman, Cytogard airflow diagram*

General comments

A carbon exhaust filter is not a true filter but a gas adsorption cell which can be subject to channelling. It can release carbon particles into the room and it is not possible to test the adsorption capacity non-destructively. There seems little need for a carbon exhaust filter, particularly if the air exhaust is ducted to the outside.

Where cabinets are sited in aseptic suites, product protection is simplified because the cabinet itself is in a Class E/F environment.[3] If situated in a dispensary or on a ward, local air turbulence will be a more critical determining factor of operator and product protection than the cabinet's design.

Of the two cabinets, the M.A.T. Cytomat appears technically superior but it is also the more expensive.

2 Isolators

Standards

There are no standards in the UK for isolators to be used for aseptic dispensing. BS 5726[1] includes a reference to Class III containment, microbiological safety cabinets.

Operating principles

Isolators are totally enclosed work stations supplied with filtered air which should meet BS 5295, Class E/F.[3] Operators use either glove ports, or a half-suit arrangement to access the working area. Materials are introduced either through an air lock or using an access port and docking device. During operation the cabinet is totally sealed from the outside. Isolators can be of a rigid or a flexible structure and their design can have a considerable impact upon their potential uses and upon operating, monitoring and disinfection procedures.

Flexible film isolators (Envair UK Ltd, La Calhene Ltd, Cambridge Isolation Technology (CIT))

The dimensions and configurations of flexible isolators are variable as there are a large number of working, bank, transfer and sterilization chambers marketed. Companies will meet the design needs of the customer.

Design characteristics Flexible film isolators have an enclosure made entirely of flexible PVC film supported on a chrome or stainless steel framework. Sizes can vary and two, three or four-glove port models, half-suit or double half-suit designs are available. Inlet and outlet air is HEPA filtered (99.997%) and the air supply can be so designed that the working environment is under positive or negative pressure. The air supply is not laminar flow and normally provides the contained unit with approximately 20 air changes per hour. Rapid transfer ports on the sides of the isolator enable enclosed containers to be locked on. In connecting the two together the lid from the container locks onto the port door. The contaminated surface of the isolator door and container lid are therefore sealed together and are not exposed to the isolator when the lid is removed to allow access to the container.

The half-suit systems offer greater flexibility and all-round movement but appear at first to be claustrophobic. The suits are double layered and are fed with an air supply which both inflates and lifts the suit so that it does not press against the operator while providing a flow of air across the face and body. By their very nature, flexible isolators are more easily damaged and require care during use.

For cytotoxic reconstitution, isolators must be under negative pressure. Extra support frames are required for this and the relative pressures may cause ingress of contaminated air if the PVC canopy is pin-holed. Monitoring procedures must be capable, therefore, of detecting pin-hole leaks.

La Calhene Ltd appear to have the more sophisticated range and they offer a wider choice of transfer containers but they are also the most expensive.

Rigid isolators

The walls of the cabinet are rigid with a totally enclosed working area. The inlet and outlet air supply is HEPA filtered (99.997%) and the air can be turbulent or laminar flow. The front panel is a clear plastic and is fitted with up to four glove ports. Materials are transferred into and out of the cabinets via air locks or enclosures.

Astecair Cytolab (Astec Environmental Systems Ltd)

Cabinet dimensions (h × w × d (mm)) 1920 × 2060 × 810; (w × d × h (mm) 2060 × 810 × 1920

Filters Five filters, comprising the system inlet and exhaust filters, the cabinet inlet and exhaust filters and the main filter. The main filter dimensions (mm) are 600 × 450 × 100.

Design characteristics The Cytolab isolator is a cast, epoxy resin, rigid construction. The front panel is a clear, acrylic glazing which can be fitted with two or four glove ports. It has a valve operated air inlet system which enables the cabinet to be operated under either positive or negative pressure. Inlet and outlet filters are located at the back of the charcoal or chemisorbent main filter. The air supply provides approximately 20 air changes per hour within the cabinet. Entry and exit ports are located on the side panel of the cabinet. These are fitted with a double door system and may be, optionally, flushed with HEPA filtered air.

Figure 2.4 shows the airflow pattern and the configuration of valves and filters within the cabinet.

Amercare Cytotoxic Drug Handling Suite (Amercare Ltd)

Dimensions (w × h × d (mm)) 2000 × 700 × 600; (w × d × h (mm)) 2000 × 600 × 700

Filters Inlet filters are cylindrical, 244 mm diameter × 305 mm long. Separate filters supply the entry enclosure and chamber. Exhaust filters are not fitted as standard but can be fitted to customer requirements.

Design characteristics This cabinet is a rigid steel construction comprising an entry/exit enclosure together with a main processing enclosure. The inlet air supply is via HEPA filters (99.997%).

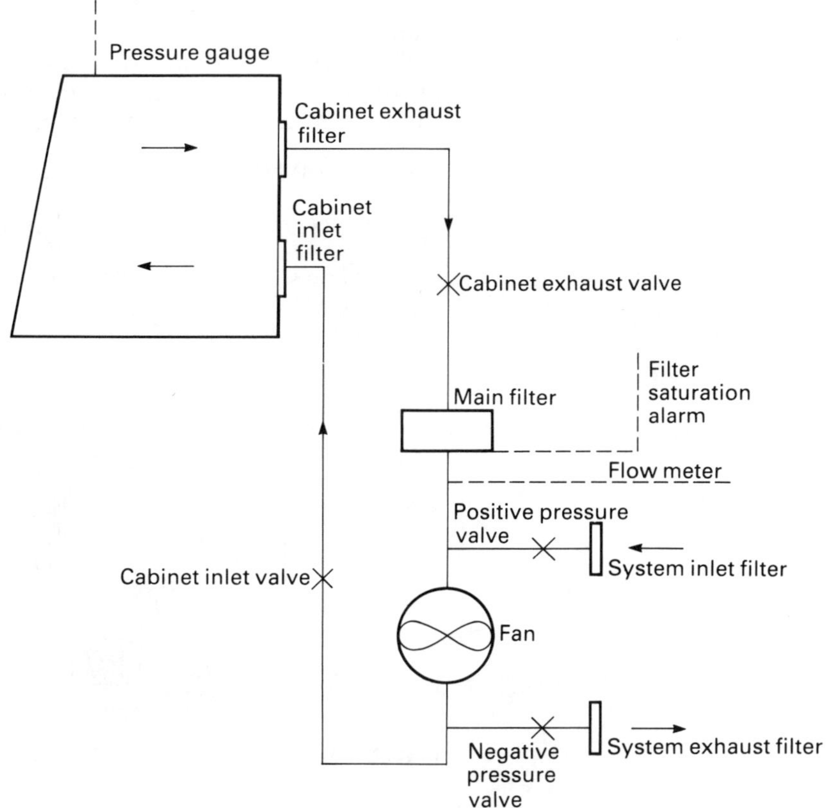

Figure 2.4: *Astec Cytolab airflow diagram*

The entry/exit enclosure is fitted at the right hand of the suite. The right hand wall of the enclosure is fitted with a vertically sliding, pneumatically-sealed door. The front face is an acrylic viewing panel with two glove ports. The left hand wall is fitted with a horizontally sliding, pneumatically-sealed door.

The processing enclosure is fitted to the left-hand side of the suite. The right-hand wall is fitted with a formed aperture to match the door in the left side of the exit/entry port. The front face is a clear acrylic panel with three glove ports. The left-hand wall of the processing unit is fitted with a bagging-out port, sealed with a removable internal bung.

Both enclosures are under negative pressure, air being drawn in via the HEPA filter located in the bench below the enclosure. The pressure is such that if the system is in any way compromised, eg by a door opening or a glove becoming damaged, air is extracted from the enclosure at a sufficient rate to give a safe inward velocity of air through the opening, allowing the negative pressure to be maintained. Air inlet and extraction is via vertical distribution tubes at the back of each enclosure. The exhaust air is ducted outside the building. The air velocity is such that it provides the cabinet with 250 air changes per hour.

The pneumatic door operating system is such that the seals on the door into the entry/exit enclosure and the door between the two enclosures are interlocked.

Figure 2.5 shows the airflow pattern in the suite.

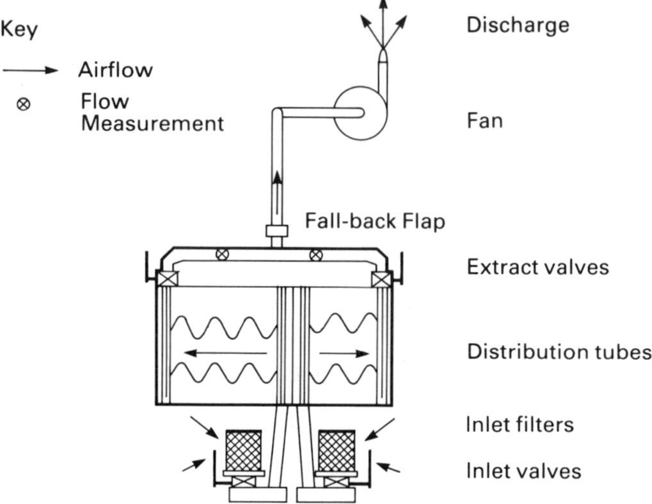

Figure 2.5: *Amercare Cytotoxic Drug Handling Suite airflow diagram*

Amercare Compact Cytotoxic Suite (Amercare Ltd)

Dimensions (w × d × h (mm)) 1600 × 600 × 700

Filters Filters are cylindrical, 244 mm diameter × 305 mm long. Exhaust filters are not fitted as standard.

Design characteristics The only difference between this unit and the Amercare Cytotoxic Drug Handling Suite is that the entry/exit enclosure is replaced by a ventilated entry/exit enclosure with no glove ports. Otherwise the operating principles of the two units are the same.

Containair Dispensing Cabinet (Envair UK)

Cabinet dimensions (w × d × h (mm)) 2432 × 695 × 1300, not including stand which is fitted to customer requirements.

Filters Downflow HEPA, 1220 mm × 508 mm × 152 mm; primary exhaust HEPA, 1130 mm × 326 mm × 203 mm; secondary exhaust HEPA, 590 mm × 460 mm × 66 mm (minipleat); hatch HEPAs, 460 mm × 320 mm × 66 mm. The exhaust filters are sealed on the upstream and downstream faces.

Design characteristics The Containair is a rigid, steel cabinet. Two glove ports are fitted into the front viewing panel which is hydraulically assisted and may be lifted to allow the installation of large pieces of equipment. The cabinet is supplied with vertical laminar flow HEPA filtered air (99.997%) and is fitted with dual exhaust HEPA filters. The air supply provides approximately 20 air changes per hour.

Transfer ports are fitted on the side panels of the cabinet and are independently flushed with HEPA filtered air.

Figure 2.6 shows the airflow pattern for the work zone. Transfer hatch ventilation is not shown.

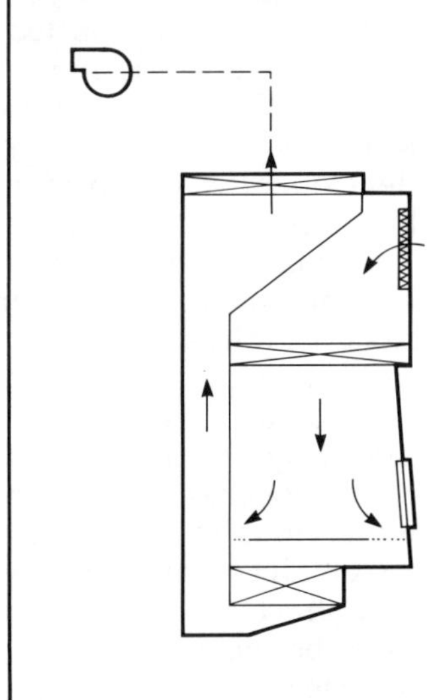

Figure 2.6: *Envair Containair airflow diagram*

General comments

Whilst the Containair cabinet is designed specifically for cytotoxic dispensing it is also suitable for aseptic dispensing as is the Astecair cabinet. The Amercare cabinets were originally designed as Radiopharmacy cabinets, and models for use in Radiopharmacy units are available. The Astecair and Containair cabinets can be adapted for radiation protection.

The rigid containment cabinets are relatively easy to clean and disinfect using hard surface disinfectants. Since they are designed to be used in an uncontrolled environment and will operate under negative pressure, high efficiency seals on all cabinet openings are essential. In this respect the design of the Amercare cabinets is superior to the other two.

In addition, those units with non-laminar air flow have dead spots within the Class E/F area[3] and purging of contaminants from the cabinets will, to a large extent, be dependent on the air turbulence created within the cabinet. The greater number of air changes in the Amercare cabinets produce a more turbulent air flow.

Sterilization of internal surfaces

Gaseous sterilization is the only practical means of sterilization of large flexible film isolators. This requires the filtered output air to be ducted outside and above the roof of the building, which adds considerably to the cost.

It is possible to link together two or more flexible isolators via the transfer ports. Components, containers and equipment can be surface sterilized, by gaseous sterilization, in one isolator overnight then transferred the following day to the adjoining isolator prior to use.

Formaldehyde and peracetic acid are the usual sterilants. Peracetic acid is reported to be the more effective and easier to use but is also the more toxic. Formaldehyde will be absorbed by the PVC and therefore time must be allowed for the gas to desorb from the canopy. Cytanox®, a gaseous sterilant developed by Cambridge Isolation Technology (CIT) is available, but there is little information on its use.

It must be stressed that gaseous sterilization cannot be recommended for the surface sterilization of articles within an isolator unless the user can fully validate the system with respect to gas desorption from packaging, closures, syringes, etc. Equally it should be noted that there is a risk of gas entry into drug or diluent containers if stress cracks are present or if the closures of individual containers are not guaranteed impervious to gas ingress.

COSHH regulations[4] would enforce the view that a safe and effective means of gas desorption, removal and disposal must be included in any sterilization equipment and protocol for use.

Sterilization of small flexible film isolators by hard surface disinfectants is not precluded but the effect of the alcoholic sprays on PVC film needs to be evaluated. Chlorhexidine-containing alcoholic sprays should be used with caution or not at all, as a film of chlorhexidine residue will build up on surfaces, potentially causing contamination of solutions.

For rigid isolators, surface disinfection with an alcoholic solution is the simplest and quickest option, but it should be noted that some manufacturers do not advocate the practice. However, direct questioning has revealed that the reservations expressed relate to long-term soaking in alcohol solutions leading to crazing of some types of clear plastic. The routine use of alcohol solutions by swab or spray application with subsequent rapid evaporation is not seen as problematic.

Astec recommend sterilization using formaldehyde gas. The gas is allowed to diffuse passively overnight and is then absorbed onto a special carbon filter the next day. The odour of formaldehyde is still detectable after this procedure. Both Amercare and Envair recommend the use of either gaseous sterilization or hard surface disinfection.

Glove ports and gauntlets (see also Chapter 3)

All isolators, whether they be rigid, flexible film or half-suit isolators, are accessed via a glove port. These are glove/sleeve arrangements which are designed to maintain the aseptic environment within the isolator. Several types of gauntlets and glove/sleeve systems, made from various materials are available and careful selection will be necessary.

Gauntlets

These are one piece, full-arm-length gloves. They are available in a range of materials. Pinholes are not uncommon since manufacturers are not always aware of the need for stringent testing for perforation during manufacturing.

They are usually changed on a weekly (or longer) basis due to the high cost, resulting in a potential risk of drug penetration and poor general hygiene, as a number of operators will use the same gloves. For these reasons, double-gloving is generally used. However, as gauntlets do not fit well, particularly under conditions of negative pressure, operator sensitivity will be reduced.

Gauntlets are usually thicker than surgeons' latex gloves, which may offset risk of drug penetration to a degree. They are not normally available pre-sterilized.

Glove/sleeve systems

These are multi-component systems consisting generally of a replaceable sleeve piece, a connecting cuff piece and the glove. The sleeve should be mechanically strong enough to remain in position without deterioration for a number of weeks. It should not be too rigid for comfortable working and should be resistant to chemical attack. The cuff piece should allow an easy, safe, aseptic glove change-over.

The glove/sleeve system allows gloves of an appropriate specification, particularly with respect to perforations and pinholes, to be used. It will, if correctly designed, allow the individual operator to fit and change gloves of correct size as frequently as required and enable the glove material to be altered without jeopardy to the isolator environment. Risk of drug penetration can be minimized in this way and general hygiene is improved as each operator can fit a fresh sterile pair of gloves each time the equipment is used.

MONITORING

1 Vertical Laminar Flow Cabinets

The microbiological monitoring programme used for horizontal LFCs can be used also for vertical LFCs. Particle counts and filter challenge tests are also similar but, in addition, operator protection factors should be regularly monitored using the KI discus apparatus.[1]

2 Isolators

Microbiological monitoring of isolators will be, in general, the same as that used for LFCs. Particle counts and filter challenge tests are also equally applicable. There is a need to monitor for pinholes and defects in the gloves, and in the canopies of flexible isolators; so regular leak tests are also required. Double gloving is often employed and finger dabbing is practised in some units as a monitoring technique.

SUMMARY

Isolators offer significant advantages over cleanrooms for small-scale aseptic operations. They can be housed in a socially cleanroom and a minimum of gowning is required. Revenue and maintenance costs are substantially less than conventional cleanrooms. The use of rigid isolators is limited by the lack of working space for larger operations and, in some cases, the size of the air locks. However, these cabinets are very suitable for small scale operations and particularly for one-off aseptic dispensing operations, since disinfection is quick and easy and materials can be introduced very simply.

Flexible isolators address the problem of space but create other problems, such as the detection of pinholes (particularly when under negative pressure), disinfection, and loading ready for use. Ideally they need to be loaded for a complete session of work and rapid, aseptic transfer of items that have been omitted is not easy.

The problems of turbulence, due to the immediate environment or the operator, limit the effectiveness of VLFCs as cytotoxic dispensing cabinets. Isolators offer a totally enclosed work area. Aseptic transfer into and out of isolators is more complicated than for VLFCs since there is no simple front aperture. In this respect the transfer hatches of the rigid isolators have an advantage over docking ports.

Isolators should be sited within a designated room or a designated area within the Pharmacy department. When installing VLFCs and isolators with external ducting, there may be problems of filtration of the air supply to the cabinet and in balancing air pressures within the room in which the cabinet is sited. Adequate consideration should also be given to the discharge of the exhaust duct.

Gaseous sterilization should only be used on those cabinets fitted with external ducting. Those isolators which lend themselves to disinfection with hard-surface disinfectants and do not require fumigation with formaldehyde or peracetic acid, are preferred by users and allow more flexibility. Also, air locks rather than access ports are preferred.

For very large scale operations and for batch manufacturing, a traditional cleanroom may be preferable because of the flexibility it allows.

Choice of gloves and glove changing procedures are an important practical consideration and these should be thoroughly investigated before purchasing decisions are made.

It should be possible to change gloves without loss of Class E/F conditions within the isolator.

REFERENCES

1. Anon. (1979). *Specification for microbiological safety cabinets, BS 5726*. British Standards Institute, London.
2. Anon. (1982). *Cytotoxic drug safety cabinets, AS 2567*. Standards Association of Australia, Sydney.
3. Anon. (1989). *Environmental cleanliness in enclosed spaces, Parts 1, 2, 3, BS 5295*. British Standards Institute, London.
4. Anon. (1988). *The control of substances hazardous to health regulations*. HMSO, London.

Protective Clothing

INTRODUCTION

Some form of protective clothing should be worn at all times when handling cytotoxics. The degree of protection required will depend on the type of preparation facility available, the nature of the agents being handled and the extent of exposure (ie preparation, checking and transportation).

The minimum requirements for the handling of cytotoxic drugs are:

▼ laboratory overall or uniform;
▼ gloves of suitable quality.

Additional protection is required for preparation of doses in an uncontrolled environment[1]:

▼ non-absorbent armlets;
▼ plastic apron;
▼ eye protection;
▼ face mask.

Armlets and an apron should be worn in addition to standard cleanroom clothing. Armlets should also be worn when preparing drugs in an isolator cabinet as the rubber sleeves may not protect the operator from gross contamination. Designated overalls should be worn for preparatory work.

The advice of the local Health and Safety or COSHH adviser should be sought when necessary.

PROTECTIVE CLOTHING

The list of suppliers of protective clothing is not exhaustive.

1 Gowns and Cleanroom Suits

These should be made of lightweight, low-linting, disposable or conventional fabric. Cleanroom suits should include headgear and footwear made of a similar material. They should be cuffed at the wrists and ankles and should fit neatly around the face.

Suppliers include, Contamination Control Apparel Ltd, Multifabs, Kimberley-Clarke, Initial Textile Services, Micronclean, Surgikos and Molnlycke.

2 Masks

Standard surgeons' masks available from Molnlycke, Klinimask and Seward are suitable for most procedures carried out in a 'contained environment' in a cleanroom. If there is a possibility of inhalation and a drug is not handled in a 'contained environment', a suitable dust mask should be worn, eg a disposable 'Bra cup' type to BS 6016.[1] A respirator mask may be required for dealing with large-scale spills or contamination.

3 Eye protection

Eye protection to BS 2092C is required for handling cytotoxic drugs if the material is not being handled in a suitable cabinet[1]. Goggles should fully enclose the eyes to protect against dust and splashes.

4 Aprons

These provide a protective, water-resistant barrier to accidental spills or sprays. They can be ethylene oxide sterilized if required. Saranex-laminated or Tyvek aprons provide added protection for use in an uncontrolled environment (*see* Armlets). Aprons are available from most manufacturers of cleanroom clothing.

5 Armlets

Protective armlets should be worn for all cytotoxic preparation and checking procedures in addition to standard cleanroom clothing or laboratory overalls. These should be made of an impervious material which prevents penetration of cytotoxics.

Laidlaw *et al.*[2] investigated the permeability of four disposable protective-clothing materials to seven antineoplastic drugs over a four-hour period. The materials tested were Saranex-laminated Tyvek, polyethylene-coated Tyvek, non-porous Tyvek and Kaycel. All of the materials evaluated afforded protection from occupational exposure to cytotoxic drugs, whereas standard gowns were completely absorbent. Saranex-laminated Tyvek and polyethylene-coated Tyvek afforded almost complete protection from the drugs. Non-porous Tyvek or Kaycel did allow some drug permeation, although the maximum permeation over a four-hour exposure time was 3.3% of the applied drug dose.

As a general recommendation it is suggested that Saranex-laminated or polyethylene-coated Tyvek armlets should be worn over standard cleanroom clothing for preparation of cytotoxics in a VLFC where the arms of the operator are exposed throughout. These armlets should also be worn when preparing cytotoxics in an isolator cabinet as the rubber sleeves may not protect the operator from gross contamination (*see* gloves in Chapter 2, Facilities). Non-porous Tyvek armlets would be suitable for all other preparation and checking procedures.

Suitable armlets are available from Micronclean and Contamination Control Apparel Ltd.

6 Gloves

Disposable gloves should be worn at all times when preparing and checking cytotoxics.

The suitability of a wide range of commercially available gloves for cytotoxic handling has been investigated.[3-7] No gloves were completely impermeable to all cytotoxics. Glove material, thickness and integrity were the major factors affecting drug permeation.

Recommendations vary as to which type of glove material (latex, rubber or PVC) provides best protection. Thomas and Fenton-May[4] found that the permeation rate of carmustine varied with glove material and glove thickness and that some gloves made from each of the three materials afforded adequate protection. When selecting gloves for use with cytotoxics, the user must be assured that the glove material is of a suitable thickness and integrity to maximize protection. Manufacturers should be asked to supply information on thickness and durability. The use of poor quality, cheap gloves is neither cost-effective nor safe because multiple glove changes are required to ensure integrity.

It has been suggested that operatives should double-glove and change the gloves every 30 minutes.[1] In practice, provided gloves which assure adequate protection are worn and are changed at the end of each work session, immediately following known contact with a cytotoxic, or if punctured, double-gloving should not be necessary. However, it should be standard practice when dealing with major spillages and when handling carmustine, mustine, amsacrine and thiotepa. Double-gloving is recommended for isolators because not all gauntlets are impermeable to cytotoxics (*see* Chapter 2, Facilities for details of Isolator gloves).

REFERENCES

1. Glass, D.C. *et al.* (1989). *The control of substances hazardous to health. Guidance for the initial assessment in hospitals.* HMSO, London.
2. Laidlaw, J.L. *et al.* (1985). Permeability of four disposable protective-clothing materials to seven antineoplastic drugs. *Am. J. Hosp. Pharm.* **42**, 2449–2454.
3. Oldcorne, M.A. *et al.* (1987). Handling cytotoxic drugs. *Pharm. J.* **238**, 488.
4. Thomas, P.H. and Fenton-May V. (1987). Protection offered by various gloves to carmustine exposure. *Pharm. J.* **238**, 775–777.
5. Slevin, M.L. *et al.* (1984). The efficiency of protective gloves used in the handling of cytotoxic drugs. *Cancer Chem. and Pharm.* **12**, 151–153.
6. Laidlaw, J.L. *et al.* (1984). Permeability of latex and polyvinyl chloride gloves to 20 antineoplastic drugs. *Am. J. Hosp. Pharm.* **41**, 2618–2623.
7. Anon. (1987). Working party report – guidelines for the handling of cytotoxic drugs: amendment. *Pharm. J.* **238**, 414.

CHAPTER 4

Disposables

INTRODUCTION

Despite the range of items available for drug reconstitution, transport and disposal, the overriding aim when selecting disposables for use with cytotoxic drugs should be suitability, safety and simplicity. Devices listed in this chapter meet all three criteria, although choice of particular items will depend on the level of service provided. The cost of many of the devices may seem prohibitive but their use can be justified for health and safety reasons. Most hospital Supplies departments stock a wide range of disposables.

SYRINGES AND ADMINISTRATION SYSTEMS

It is recommended that syringes used for cytotoxic drugs be luer-lock and made of polypropylene, as the material is chemically inert.[1,2] Styrene syringes are specifically not recommended for cytotoxic drugs. In certain instances, manufacturers recommend a specific type of syringe be used for a particular product, eg amsacrine. Standards for syringes are given in BS 5081, part 1 (1987)[3] and ISO 7886.[4]

Brands of syringes currently recommended for use with cytotoxic drugs include Becton Dickinson, Plastipak; Sherwood Medical, Monoject; B.Braun, Omnifix, Injekt and Perfusor and Terumo. This list is not exhaustive and other brands may be suitable, subject to testing.

Syringes are usually made in three parts – the barrel and piston of plastic materials and the plunger of rubber (Figure 4.1). Certain grades of rubber have been found to release water-soluble materials on prolonged contact with drug solutions.[5,6] Hence, chemical interactions between rubber extractives and the drugs are possible. If it is intended to store drugs in a particular brand of syringe for prolonged periods, it is advisable to check that there is no such interaction. B.Braun make a polypropylene two-piece syringe with no rubber plunger which overcomes the possibility of an interaction between plunger and drug.

In addition to ensuring that a drug is stable on storage, it is necessary to check that there is not an unacceptable degree of water loss from the syringe. So far, the syringes made by B.Braun and Becton Dickinson have been tested and found to be satisfactory regarding water loss.[7] It is recommended that

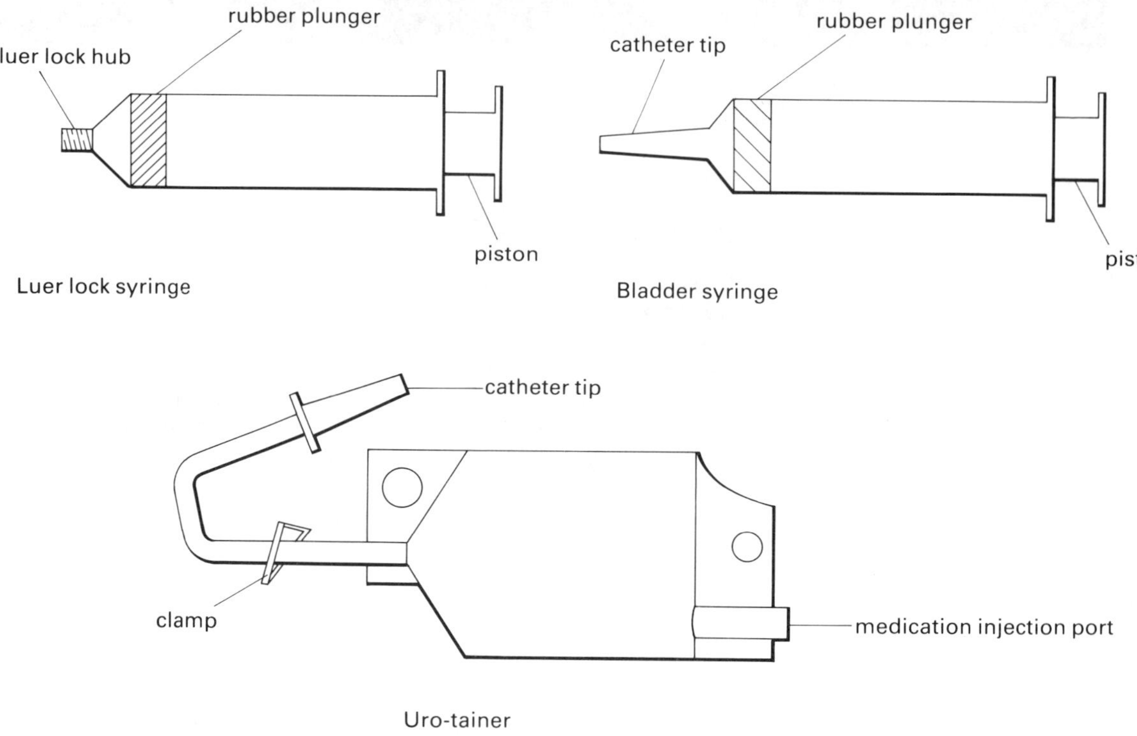

Figure 4.1: *Disposable administration systems*

this test be carried out at 37°C, to provide a 'worst case', 2–8°C and under ambient conditions. It is advisable to carry out the tests with syringes that have been over-wrapped.

Syringes must be fitted with blind hub closures, not needles, when prepared in the Pharmacy. The blind hubs should be luer-lock, must be a good fit and not permit leakage, and must be easy for medical and nursing staff to remove safely. Blind hubs suitable for use with cytotoxic drugs include those made by Becton Dickinson and B.Braun.

Bladder instillations of cytotoxic drugs are better presented in bladder syringes or Uro-tainers (Figure 1). Many bladder syringes have luer-lock connections in addition to the usual catheter tip. However, the addition of a luer-lock fitting to a bladder irrigation container may be potentially hazardous as it could facilitate IV administration of the bladder irrigation solution. Uro-tainers (Clinimed Ltd) are pre-filled devices specifically made for the instillation of fluids into the bladder. The most useful of the range, from the point of view of cytotoxic drug dispensing, is the Uro-tainer M, which contains 50 ml or 100 ml of 0.9% sodium chloride solution. It has the advantage of an additive port so that drugs can be added to the solution.

NEEDLES AND FILTRATION SYSTEMS

1 Needles

When removing solutions from vials or ampoules, it is essential to use as wide a bore needle as possible to prevent undue pressure building up in the system. This is particularly important with viscous solutions such as etoposide. Specifications for needles are included in BS 5081, part 1 (1987)[3] and ISO 7886.[4] The length of the needle used will depend on the nature of the procedure being carried out.

Specialized transfer needles include the Becton Dickinson needles for drawing up and reconstituting medications. Both the Trans 18 and Nokor Admix needles reduce the risk of producing cores of rubber from vial caps.

Abbott, Butterfly needles, which consist of a winged needle attached to a length of tubing with a luer-lock connector at the end, are useful for multiple additions or withdrawals from infusion bags or vials. They are available in standard needle sizes.

2 Filtration Systems

Sterilizing filters are not recommended for use with solutions of cytotoxic drugs because of the risk of pressurizing the system (*see* section on Air Vents). If a solution requires clarification, a filter with a pore size of not less than 5 μm can be used but with great caution. Filter needles are available from Becton Dickinson, Sherwood Medical and B.Braun. Filter straws or quills are fitted with a flexible tube rather than a needle and are useful for drawing up solutions from ampoules. The rate of flow is greater than with a needle. Examples include the B.Braun, Filter Straw and the Avon Medical (Smith and Nephew), Filter Kwill with 10 μm filter. (NB Filters are not recommended for use with etoposide as there is a potential chemical interaction with the material of which most filters are made.)

RECONSTITUTION DEVICES AND AIR VENTS

1 Reconstitution Devices

A number of reconstitution devices are available, but not all are suitable for use with cytotoxic drugs. The devices have either a short, fine plastic spike or a wide bore needle. Spikes can make large holes in rubber bungs, with the possibility of leakage of the solution from around the spike. In addition, there is a risk of producing a 'core' of rubber. Needles are less likely to compromise the integrity of the rubber and are more suitable for use in the reconstitution of cytotoxic drugs than spikes.

Suitable products include the Sherwood, Monoject Medication Transfer Needle, the Baxa Intravenous Additive Transfer Needle and the Baxter Healthcare Viaflex, Drug Reconstitution Device. These three products are non-vented and have no filter. The Baxter device is only suitable for vials with a bung diameter greater than 20 mm. B.Braun produce a double-ended filter transfer needle but like the others it is non-vented.

Several special withdrawal devices are available with short, fine plastic spikes. They are designed to simplify the aspiration of measured volumes of diluent or drug from multi-dose containers, by syringe. Examples include the Viggo, FloPro Withdrawal Cannula and the B.Braun, Sterifix Mini-Spike. Both have a 5 µm air filter which prevents negative pressure in the vial and are available with an in-line 5 µm solution filter. International Medication Systems (UK), make a variety of withdrawal devices including the Bag-A-Jet, which is used to decant fluid from an infusion bag. This may be useful when it is necessary to withdraw fluid from an infusion bag prior to the addition of a drug.

2 Air Vents

The hazard of aerosol production during the preparation of cytotoxic drugs is well recognized. To prevent the risk of exposure to individuals carrying out preparation, 'air venting' of drug vials is recommended before reconstitution.[1,2,8] This can be carried out in one of three ways: using an air vent; a hydrophobic filter-needle unit, or a negative pressure procedure. The negative pressure procedure described by Wilson and Solimando eliminates the need for venting.[9] However, it requires consistent, impeccable technique, which some operatives find difficult to maintain. Hydrophobic filter-needle units are relatively expensive but it is prudent to balance cost with increased safety to the individual.

Devices on the market which have short fine plastic spikes are not recommended, except where supplied by the manufacturer for a particular product, because of the potential for leakage around the spike and rubber bung of the vial.

Suitable air vents include the Baxa, Venting Pins, which are available in two needle sizes and two filter sizes, and the Avon Medical (Smith and Nephew), Air Inlet Set, which has a valve and non-wetting filter combination. The Avon, Air Inlet Set is long with a wide-bore needle making it difficult to use with smaller vials.

Another means of reducing aerosol formation is the Medema Safety Bag (Cambmac Instruments Ltd) which traps the aerosol in a sterile bag attached to a needle venting the vial. Its main disadvantage is that it is very cumbersome to use.

Hydrophobic filter-needle units include the Millex-25 Vent Filter Unit (Millipore) and the Cytosafe Needle (Baxa) (Figure 4.2). The Millex-25, Vent Filter Unit consists of a needle attached to a 0.2 µm hydrophobic membrane filter in a plastic housing. It can be difficult to use with smaller vials as both the filter unit and the needle of the reconstituting syringe need to be accommodated in the rubber bung of the vial. The Cytosafe is a 19 gauge non-coring needle with a venting system incorporating a 0.2 µm hydrophobic filter.

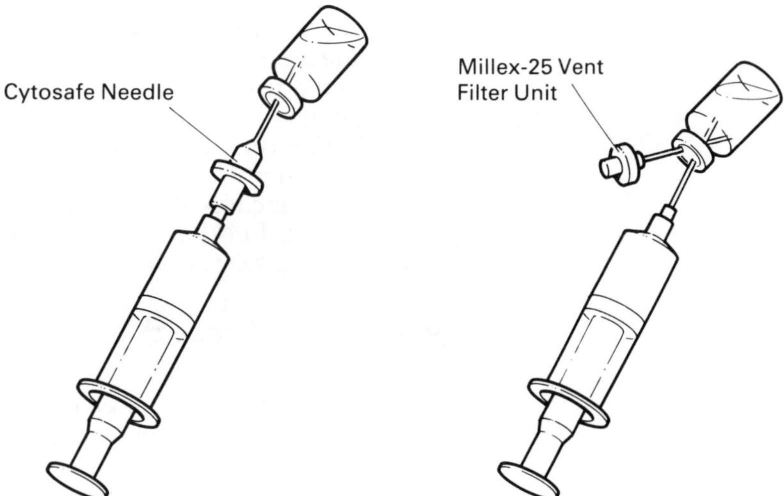

Figure 4.2: *Comparison of hydrophobic filter-needle units*

It is available in two needle lengths, 18 mm and 47 mm, to accommodate all vial and bottle sizes. It has a luer-lock connection which can be attached directly to the syringe used for reconstituting the drug.

INCIDENTAL ITEMS

1 Cleaning Equipment

All cleaning equipment should only be used in the designated aseptic area. Any cloths, sponges or mop-heads can be used provided they are low-lint and autoclavable. It may be cheaper to buy unsterile cloths or mop-heads and use in-house sterilizing facilities if available. If there are several areas to be cleaned, the use of colour coding might be applicable.

Manufacturers of cleaning equipment suitable for use include Contamination Control Apparel Ltd, Micronclean Ltd and Scott Young Service Systems Ltd.

2 Trays

These can be used for many purposes, including collection of waste inside an isolator or VLFC, as a confined environment for cytotoxic drug reconstitution and for setting-up each preparation prior to reconstitution. They come in a variety of materials (eg plastic and foil) and sizes. It is important that they can be easily cleaned or sterilized depending on their use.

Examples include foil trays from Lakeland Plastics and plastic trays from Henleys Medical Supplies Ltd.

3 Absorbent Mats

These are used for lining working surfaces. Their use in VLFCs is not ideal because recirculation of air is hampered, but they may have a use in isolators. Their ease of disposal once contaminated is an advantage. Any absorbent material of suitable size can be used provided it can be sterilized for use within an aseptic area.

Examples include Benchkote Surface Protectors (Whatman Labsale Ltd), Luckham Bench Shield and Sterile, Micron Foamwipes (Micronclean Ltd).

4 Ampoule Snappers

These are useful to avoid contamination with glass splinters. They are supplied free of charge with some drugs. Sepha Products make a reusable ampoule snapper, Clic'Open.

5 Oddments

Items such as three-way taps (stopcocks) and intermittent infusion plugs are available from hospital Sterile Supplies departments.

PACKAGING, TRANSPORT AND DISPOSAL

Packaging and transportation systems for cytotoxics must provide adequate physical, chemical and light protection for the drug during storage and transportation; be relatively impervious to the atmosphere; be robust; be tamperproof; provide adequate protection to the handler; contain any leaked solution and allow easy identification of the contained drugs throughout.

For general guidance on the disposal of cytotoxic drugs and materials contaminated with them, refer to Chapter 6. Equipment used for disposal should comply with the requirements for packaging and transport.

1 Tamper-evident Seals

The injection ports of infusion bags and the tops of infusion bottles (eg treosulfan) should ideally be sealed after addition of a drug or reconstitution. This prevents the further addition of drugs and indicates any loss of integrity during storage and transport.

Devices suitable for use include the Baxa, IVA Seal III, sterile seals for IV bags, vials and bottles, the Baxa, Inject-Lock port saver, and Baxter Healthcare, additive cap for IV bags.

2 Packaging

All cytotoxic preparations should be packed in leak-proof containers after preparation. Polythene tubing which can be heat sealed to give an air/water tight seal and which can be cut to enclose any size or shape of container is recommended. Grip top bags should be avoided as the seal is easily broken. Opaque polythene can be used for drugs requiring light protection; however this generally needs to be ordered as a 'special' item and is more expensive than clear polythene. These double as light protection covers on the ward. Polythene of gauge 200–250 g is suitable for most purposes; however 500 g polythene may be required for outer-packaging of items being transported to off-site centres.

Layflat polythene tubing is available from G W Heath & Co Ltd, Transatlantic Plastics Ltd, Tavak Ltd, Lakeland Plastics and C A Swain Ltd.

Heat sealers are available from a number of sources. The sealer selected must create an adequate seal and must be durable enough to endure repeated use. Domestic heat sealers are not suitable for the grades of plastic recommended.

Heat sealers are available from Hulme Martin Ltd, Tavak Ltd and Transatlantic Plastics Ltd.

3 Protective Packaging and Transportation Devices

Cytotoxics may be transported to wards and clinics in any of the standard hospital delivery containers, provided these will protect the agents from damage; will contain any possible leakage; will ensure the stability of the contained drug and are tamperproof. Cytotoxics should not be transported in the same container as other drugs and the nature of the contained packages should be clearly indicated on the outer container.

For transportation to other hospitals and for use in the community, packaging requirements are more stringent. Specialist transportation systems (Envopak Ltd) may be purchased or suitable systems may be designed using standard protective packaging.

4 Sharps Containers

Sharps containers should be robust enough to contain any leaked solutions and sharps. Ideally, they should be constructed of plastic rather than lined cardboard with tight fitting lids which can be sealed when the container is full. Absorbent material (paper towel or absorbent granules) should be placed in the bottom of the containers to mop up leaked solutions. The containers should be brightly coloured with space to indicate the nature of the contents both during use and whilst awaiting disposal. Most manufacturers can supply a range of sizes for use in isolators, cleanrooms and on the ward.

It is essential to carry out quality assurance on all new types of sharps box and to check that they are suitable for use in standard incinerators.

REFERENCES

1. Anon. (1983). Guidelines for the handling of cytotoxic drugs – working party report. *Pharm. J.* **230**, 230–231.
2. Anon. (1983). *The safe handling of cytotoxic drugs.* ASTMS, Health and Safety Office, Special Report.
3. Anon. (1987). *Sterile hypodermic syringes and needles, Part 1 Specification of sterile hypodermic syringes for single use. BS 5081.* British Standards Institute, London.
4. Anon. (1984). *Sterile hypodermic syringes for single use. ISO 7886.* (Available through the Standards Institute of the relevant country.)
5. Petersen, M.C. *et al.* (1981). Leaching of 2-(2-hydroxyethyl-mercapto) benzothiazole into contents of disposable syringes. *J. Pharm. Sci.* **70**, 1139–1143.
6. Reepmeyer, J.C. and Juhl, Y.H. (1983). Contamination of injectable solutions with 2-mercaptobenzothiazole leached from rubber closures. *J. Pharm. Sci.* **72**, 1302–1305.
7. Parkinson, R. *et al.* (1989). Stability of low-dose heparin in pre-filled syringes. *Brit. J. Pharm. Prac.* **11**, 34–36.
8. Stolar, M.H. *et al.* (1983). Recommendations for handling cytotoxic drugs in hospitals. *Am. J. Hosp. Pharm.* **40**, 1163–1171.
9. Wilson, J.P. and Solimando, D.A. (1981). Aseptic technique as a safety precaution in the preparation of antineoplastic agents. *Hosp. Pharm.* **16**, 575–581.

CHAPTER 5

Ambulatory Infusion Pumps for Cytotoxic Therapy

INTRODUCTION

Traditionally, cytotoxic chemotherapy has been administered in single or combined regimens which have been designed to maximize cell-kill whilst minimizing toxicity. However, in practice, these high dose, 'pulsed' regimens are not ideal because of the need to hospitalize the patients and the high incidence of side-effects which can delay further therapy.

Growing evidence has shown that continuous infusion of a low-dose of a cytotoxic drug achieves equivalent or higher tumour concentrations over a longer period than bolus, pulsed therapy.[1] The rational for low-dose continuous infusion therapy is discussed in more detail in Chapter 10.

In response to the demand for this method of administration, there have been rapid advances in pump technology. A wide variety of ambulatory infusion pumps are now available, ranging in complexity from external syringe drivers to implantable, programmable pumps.

The pumps described are those available in the UK. A larger range of pumps are available worldwide and readers are directed to the literature available in their own country for details of other types of pump which have been used for the administration of cytotoxic chemotherapy.

Readers are also referred to Chapter 10 for further information on the Graseby syringe driver and details of the Parker Micropump which have been used in the HOPE programme.[2]

SYRINGE PUMPS

Model: Braun Medical, Perfusor M (Figure 5.1); Graseby, MS16A (Figure 5.2) and MS26; Critikon, Syringe Minder 2.

Syringe pumps are pocket-sized, usually battery-operated and are simple in design with only a few alarms eg low battery, end of infusion and occlusion pressure. They use a range of syringes from 1 ml to 35 ml, although individual models may be limited to a narrower range.

The drug reservoir is a pre-filled syringe which is firmly clamped onto the pump. The pump is driven by a small battery-powered motor, or, in the case of the Braun, Perfusor M, by a clockwork mechanism. A rotating lead screw (or drive shaft) moves the actuator (or drive nut)

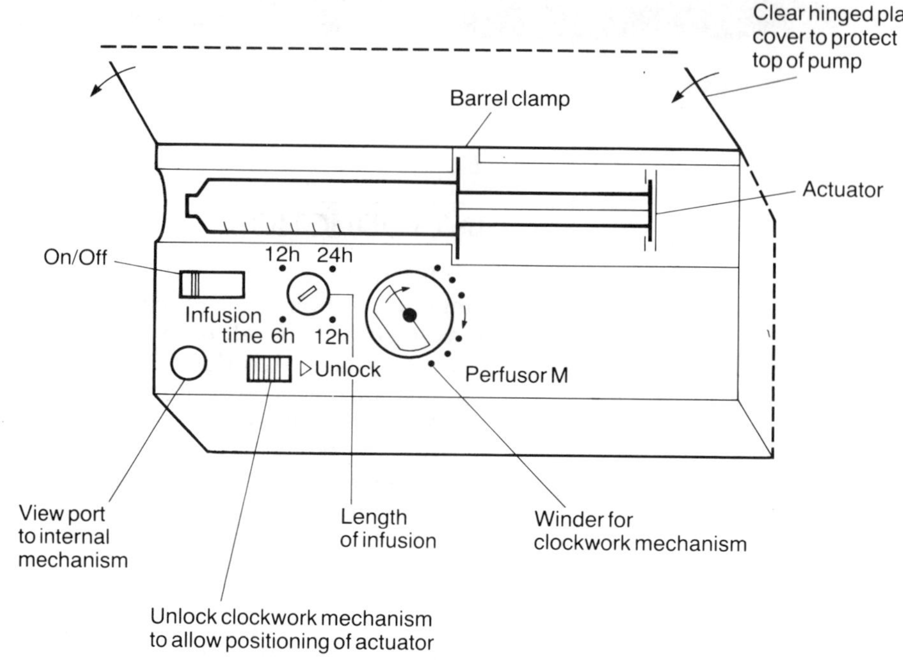

Figure 5.1: *Braun Medical Perfusor M. Pump*

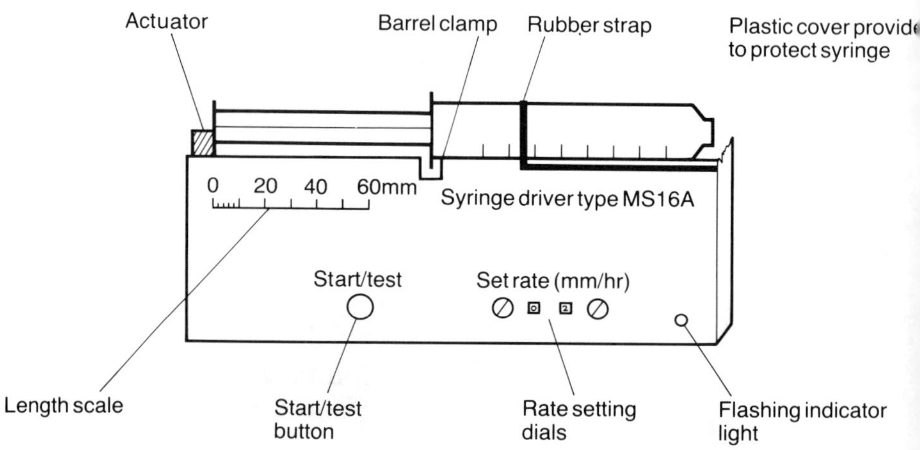

Figure 5.2: *Graseby MS16A Pump*

down the device at a constant rate, pushing the syringe plunger into the syringe barrel. The delivery rate of the drug is determined by the diameter of syringe and the speed at which the lead screw rotates.

Syringe pumps have been used successfully for self-administration of IV antibiotics[3] and cytotoxic agents.[4] They can be used with variable flow rates to a high level of accuracy

(+/− 2% to 5%). Due to the pressure generated, the pump can be used for both intra-arterial and intravenous infusions. The syringe size is a limiting factor and, if larger volumes are required, it is necessary to replace the syringe reservoir several times.

To set up the pumps, the administration line is primed either manually, before putting the syringe in the pump, or by a venting mechanism, if included in the pump. Priming should be carried out prior to rate setting in pumps that use the mm/hr or mm/day system, since at low infusion rates the dead volume of the tubing could alter the final infusion time by several hours. The syringe is placed into the pump and fixed in position. The actuator should be placed as close to the plunger as possible, to ensure that there is a little slack to take up in the lead screw when the pump is started. If the priming procedure or positioning of the actuator are not performed correctly, then, at low infusion rates, this could result in no drug being delivered for up to an hour and the patency of the venous access may be compromised.

The infusion rates are calculated in mm/hr for the Graseby, MS16A and Syringe Minder 2 pumps or mm/day for the Graseby, MS26 pump. Errors can occur when changing the pump setting if the patient or user does not understand the concept of mm/hr instead of ml/hr; or alternatively, confuses hours with days. The Syringe Minder 2 pump has preset rates of travel, 1, 2, 3, 4, 5, 6, 8, 10, 11, 12 mm/hr. The Graseby, MS16A and MS26 have continuously variable rates which are set as required. The Braun, Perfusor M has three preset rates of travel which deliver the contents of a 10 ml syringe in 6, 12 or 24 hr.

All of the pumps have a fixed occlusion pressure which causes the pump to alarm or stop. However, due to the need to overcome the build-up of pressure when infusing viscous fluids, the pressure at which the pump will alarm can be high. At low flow rates there is a considerable delay before the alarm is activated. This problem has been overcome in larger infusion pumps by positioning a pressure sensing device in the extension set rather than in the pump, but this feature is not yet available on the ambulatory pumps.

Patient education and training are required to ensure correct rate setting, mounting of syringe and priming of the set. They also need to be aware of the various alarms and how to deal with resulting malfunctions. Some knowledge is required of the mechanism of the syringe pumps. Checks must be kept on the batteries.

ELASTOMERIC PUMPS

Model: Baxter Infusor (Figure 5.3)

This is a novel delivery system which employs elastomer technology for drug delivery. The balloon, which acts as both drug reservoir and the pump, is made of an inert polyisoprene

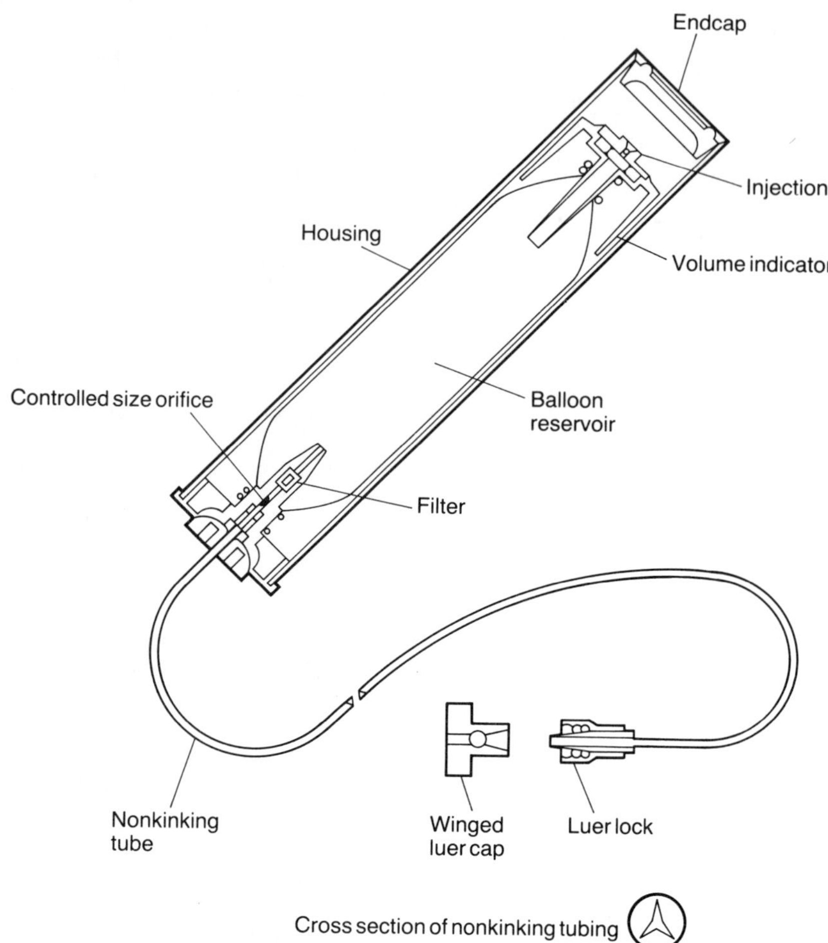

Figure 5.3: *Baxter Infusor Pump*

rubber material. This gives it elastic properties enabling the reservoir, once expanded, to contract back to its original shape and size.

The operating principle of the pump is the Hagen-Poiseville Law[5] which states that flow through a tube is a function of pressure difference (P), radius of the lumen (r), length of the tube (l), and viscosity of the liquid (v).

The law is represented by the equation

$$F = \frac{P \times \pi r^4}{8 \times v \times l}$$

The variable function is viscosity, which will be affected by vehicle and temperature. The effects of the vehicle are known if glucose or 0.9% sodium chloride solution are used[6] and temperature fluctations are kept to a minimum by wearing the Infusor close to the skin. High concentrations of drugs occasionally affect viscosity.

The drug solution is filled aseptically into the balloon reservoir to a maximum volume of 60 µl. Of this 60 µl volume, 48 µl is usually infused over 24 hours, leaving a 12 µl reserve to maintain venous patency in case the patient is unable to replace the Infusor at the normal time. It is important that there are no air bubbles in the balloon. The balloon reservoir inflates to create a sustained internal pressure of approximately 490 mmHg. A rubber septum seals the unit when the filling needle is withdrawn. The administration set of microbore tubing is automatically primed in about 15 minutes.

The patient removes the winged luer cap from the administration set and attaches the Infusor to his venous access device. The drug is delivered via a 10 µm filter at a constant rate of 2 ml/hr (diluent 5% glucose solution) or 2.2 ml/hr (diluent 0.9% sodium chloride solution). The duration of infusion can be altered by adjusting the volume filled and dosage can be altered by adjusting the volume or drug concentration. The Infusor can be used by the intra-arterial or intravenous route.

The Baxter Infusor is intended for single use and is not designed to be refilled or resterilized for repeat use. Therefore, although there is no capital cost involved in the pump, since it cannot be reused, revenue costs are high. The Infusor is light (100 g filled), small (16 cm long), comfortable in use and silent in operation. It is provided with a fabric holder which is pinned inside the patient's clothes.

The Infusor has been studied in 18 patients who received 52 treatment courses, representing 247 patient-days of treatment at home rather than in hospital. During this period there was no known failure to infuse and no reported flow rate or administration difficulties. There was one report of a leaking unit.[6]

The Infusor has been used to administer a number of drugs including morphine,[7] heparin,[8] cyclophosphamide, fluorouracil, doxorubicin, methotrexate, vincristine and vinblastine.

Table 5.1: Stability of cytotoxic drugs in the Infusor device

Drug	Vehicle	Conc (mg/ml)	Temp (°C)	'Stable' for (days)
Cyclophosphamide	0.9% saline	2–20	2–8	48
			RT	2
Doxorubicin	0.9% saline	0.2–1.0	2–8	30
			RT	2
Methotrexate	0.9% saline	1.12–12.5	2–8	105
			RT	2
Fluorouracil	5% glucose, 0.9% saline	5–50	RT	15
Vincristine	0.9% saline	0.2	2–8	51
			RT	2
Vinblastine	0.9% saline	0.015–0.5	2–8	21

RT = room temperature (usually 25°C)

There are no published data on stability or compatibility of these injections in the device. The information in Table 1 is based upon research that has been conducted by Baxter Healthcare Ltd and made available in a brochure, but full details are not yet available for scientific evaluation. The parameters under which stability is considered to be satisfactory have not been fully described. This information should, therefore, be considered for guidance purposes only. It has not been included in the relevant Drug Monographs.

The patient needs to be educated about storage, infusion rates, monitoring the infusion and care of his central line after completion of the infusion. The Infusor is popular with patients in comparison with more sophisticated pumps[1] because they do not have to be concerned with battery checks, setting of infusion rates or monitoring for mechanical malfunction of the pump. In addition, as the unit is disposable, they do not have equipment to return to the hospital at the end of treatment.

PERISTALTIC PUMPS

Model: Pharmacia/Deltec, CADD-1 (Figure 5.4)

This pump employs a motorized rotating drum, powered by a battery, which rolls over a silicone tube. The drug reservoir is a 50 ml or 100 ml disposable bag. It is more sophisticated than the other pumps discussed since it is programmable and the infusion rate and drug dose can be varied. The CADD-1 has six alarms comprising: internal malfunction; set up review; pump stopped; lower residual volume in medication cassette; low battery and occlusion. There are a number of lock levels for varying patient involvement in the programming of the dose and rate of infusion. Although the pump is more sophisticated it aims to be user-friendly, but still requires a significant amount of training to ensure correct usage. With this in mind, the company have prepared training programmes for operators. Despite the many features the pump is compact (3 × 9 × 16 cm) and light (425 g).

Table 5.2: *Stability of cytotoxic drugs in the Deltec, CADD-1 device*

Drug	Vehicle	Conc (mg/ml)	Temp (°C)	'Stable' for (days)
Cisplatin	0.9% saline	1	25	7
Cyclophosphamide	WFI	20	4	14
Cyclophosphamide	WFI	20	35	1
Cytosine	0.9% saline	20	4	14
Cytosine	0.9% saline	20	35	10
Doxorubicin	WFI	2	37	5
Fluorouracil	–	50	25	14
Methotrexate	–	25	4	14
Methotrexate	–	25	35	7
Mitomycin	WFI	0.2	37	5

WFI = water for injection

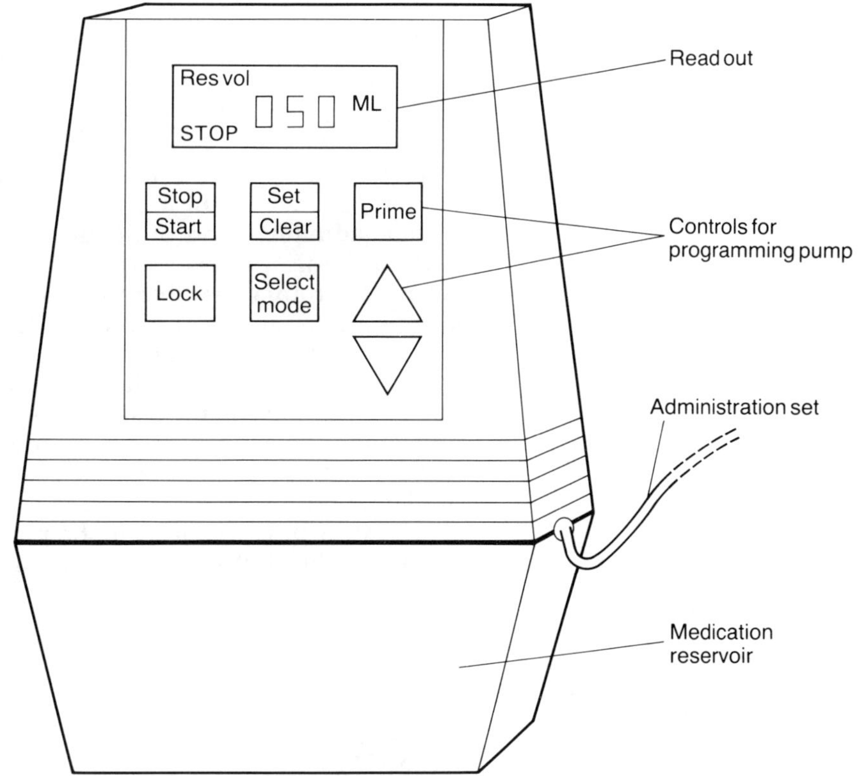

Figure 5.4: *Pharmacia/Deltec Cadd-1 Pump*

Information on the stability of various cytotoxic drugs in the device has been provided by Pharmacia. The studies were conducted at Apotekseolaget AB Central Laboratories and Apotekseolaget AB Karolinska Pharmacy, Stockholm, Sweden. It has been provided as a personal communication but details have not yet been made available for scientific evaluation. The parameters under which stability is considered have not been described. This information should, therefore, be considered for guidance purposes only. It has not been included in the relevant Drug Monographs.

IMPLANTABLE PUMPS

Models: Infusaid and Alzet

These are units that have been developed from the implanted injection port (*see* Chapter 10). Current pumps are about 10 cm in diameter with a reservoir of less than 50 ml. They are implanted in a subcutaneous pocket, which is intended to be unobtrusive but accessible to the patient.

The aim of these devices is to target therapy and decrease the severity of systemic side-effects. They are associated with a decrease in the incidence of infections at the injection port and catheter tip, compared with external pumps. A further advance is that they allow the patient greater freedom of activity. Implantable pumps have been used to deliver drugs by the intravenous, intraperitoneal, intrathecal, intra-arterial and epidural routes. In the USA their use in the intra-arterial hepatic administration of floxuridine has been reported.[9]

The Infusaid pumps consist of a drug reservoir chamber, separated from a chamber that contains a charging fluid (freon). Condensation and evaporation of freon provides the force for drug delivery through an outlet restrictor to the patient's catheter. The size of the drug reservoir differs between models (22–37 ml). Their main disadvantage is that the flow rate is set and cannot be altered. However, developments in this field aim to allow programming and changes of flow rate after implantation.

The Alzet pump is an osmotic pump that has been used in animal studies but it has only recently been investigated in humans.

CONCLUSION

A summary of the features of the ambulatory pumps discussed is contained in Table 3 (*see* opposite).

Ambulatory pumps have made the concept of continuous infusion attainable, with all the concurrent benefits previously mentioned. All the pumps provide accurate dosing and are portable. Pumps differ in the number of features available, which may include flexible administration rates, variable reservoir sizes and range of alarms. The proposed use of the pump should be considered when selecting features required. With all the pumps, not only the capital cost of the pump, but also the cost of disposables that are required for each infusion are significant factors to be considered.

For successful home treatment with ambulatory pumps, the patient must feel confident and be proficient in the use of his unit. Patient education is an important part of any ambulatory programme and the level of knowledge required and staff time involved in training and providing a back-up service for each type of pump should be carefully evaluated.

Acknowledgement

The authors would like to thank Dr J. Ford, Pharmacy Department, Liverpool Polytechnic, for helpful discussion.

Table 5.3: *Summary of pumps described*

Make/Model	Range Infusion Time	Weight	Dimensions	Pump Mechanism	Reservoir	Battery	Flow Rate and Accuracy		Alarm*
Graseby Medical									
MS16A	30 min to 60 hr	175 g	16.5×2.3×5.3 cm	syringe pump electric	2 ml–35 ml syringe	9 V	0–99 mm/hr variable	+/–5%	1, 2, 3
MS26	12 hr to 60 days	175 g	16.5×2.3×5.3 cm	syringe pump electric	2 ml–35 ml syringe	9 V	0–99 mm/day variable	+/–5%	1, 2, 3
Braun Medical									
Perfusor M	6 to 24 hr	450 g	17×7.5×3.5 cm	syringe pump clock-work	10 ml Braun Omnifix syringe	none	10 ml in 6–24 hr fixed	+/–5%	none
Critikon									
Syringe Minder 2	4 to 50 hr	185 g (250 g in case)	11.7×5×1 cm	syringe pump electric	2 ml–20 ml syringe	9 V	1–12 mm/hr fixed intervals	+/–3%	1, 2, 3
Pharmacia/Deltec									
CADD 1	1 hr to 5 days	425 g	2.8×9×16 cm	peristaltic rotary pro-grammable	50 ml/ 100 ml cassette	9 V	0–299 ml/day	theor. +/– 10% in studies +/– 3%	1, 2, 3 4, 5, 6
Baxter									
Infusor	1 to 24 hr	100 g	16.5×3 cm dia	elastomeric pressure	60 ml	none	approx 2 ml/hr	– –	none

*Alarms

1 – end of travel/infusion
2 – low battery
3 – occlusion

4 – internal malfunction
5 – lower residual volume in medication cassette
6 – start-up review (power up)

REFERENCES

1. Moody, D.G. (1986). External ambulatory infusion devices and the oncology patient. *J. Pharm. Tech*. **2**, 160–165.
2. Sewell, G.J. *et al.* (1987). HOPE for cancer. *J. Dist. Nurs.* April, 4–6.
3. Johnston, J.B. and Davidson, M.R. (1984). Use of mini-infusor syringe pump for the self-administration of IV antibiotics in the home. *Natl. Intravenous Ther. Assoc. USA*. **7**, 381–383.
4. Adams, P.S. *et al.* (1987). Pharmaceutical aspects of home infusion therapy for cancer patients. *Pharm. J.* **238**, 476–478.
5. Thomas, M. (1985). Miniaturized continuous delivery systems for injectable solutions: individual patient control and physio-chemical properties. *Proc. of the Guild*, **19**, 3–37.
6. Akahoshi, M.P. *et al.* (1987). Safety and reliability of the Travenol Infusor in administering chemotherapy in the home. *J. Pharm. Tech*. **3**, 65–68.
7. Wermeling, D.P. *et al.* (1987). Evaluation of a disposable non-electric patient-controlled analgesia device for post-operative pain. *Clin. Phar.* **6**, 307–315.
8. Merrigan, D.M. *et al.* (1987). Continuous heparin infusion in the home-bound ambulatory patient using the Travenol Infusor. *Natl. Intravenous Ther. Assoc. USA*. **10**, 122–126.
9. Kwan, J.W. (1989). High technology IV infusion devices. *Am. J. Hosp. Pharm.* **46**, 320–335.

CHAPTER 6

Health and Safety Aspects of Cytotoxic Services

INTRODUCTION

It is now well recognized that most cytotoxics are potentially hazardous substances, since they are either mutagenic, teratogenic or carcinogenic. There is also substantial evidence to show that patients may develop secondary neoplasms as a result of treatment with cancer chemotherapeutic agents,[1,2] indicating the potential threat to the health of any persons exposed to the drugs. Such risks may be acceptable for patients with life-threatening diseases but they are clearly not acceptable to hospital personnel who are exposed to such chemicals in the work-place. There is accumulating evidence that healthcare personnel involved in the preparation and manipulation of cytotoxics can absorb potentially harmful quantities of such compounds, as indicated by mutagenicity testing of blood and urine. Much of this evidence is mounting from epidemiological studies of nurses, pharmacists and pharmacy technicians. For example, recent studies have associated spontaneous abortions and malformations in the offspring of nurses with occupational exposure to cytotoxic agents.[3,4]

Nurses handling these drugs have shown increased mutagenic activity in their urine as compared with unexposed personnel.[5,6,7] Similar patterns have also been reported in the serum of oncology nurses.[8,9,10] As a result of these early studies, a number of safety measures were introduced to protect personnel handling cytotoxics. A number of studies have now been completed which highlight the fact that these improvements can substantially reduce staff exposure levels. For example, improved care in handling has been shown to reduce mutagenic activity detected in nurses' urine.[6,11] Cooke *et al.*[12] also reported that blood samples from pharmacy staff handling cytotoxics in suitably designed units showed no greater evidence of mutagenicity than unexposed controls. In a comparative study, Kolmodin-Hedman *et al.*[13], showed that the provision of adequate safety precautions significantly reduced the mutagenic activity in urine of staff in oncology units and Pharmacies. Finally, Ferguson *et al.*[14] recently reported that a group of pharmacists working in a fully-protected environment preparing cytotoxic injections did not show evidence of drug absorption, although it was noted that an occasional individual showed evidence of exposure.

There are now sufficient reports to indicate that staff working in Pharmacies who prepare cytotoxic injections for administration, or nurses working in Oncology departments, either preparing drugs for administration or dealing with patients' urine or other contaminated fluids, are potentially at risk. This risk is sufficient to indicate, unequivocally, that all necessary measures should be adopted to protect these staff from occupational exposure. It is not possible to establish maximum safe exposure levels; so all recognized steps need to be taken to prevent, or at least reduce to a minimum, exposure to these hazardous substances in the work-place. As all approaches available are, by the nature of the problem, of an indirect form, many different aspects of service operation must be included to ensure adequate, state-of-the-art, staff protection. These should include the following:

▼ staff monitoring by Occupational Health Services;
▼ provision of adequate protective environments such as safety cabinets;
▼ effective written procedures and on-going staff training;
▼ regular application of service audits;
▼ adequate procedures for dealing with spillages and disposal of all contaminated materials.

Another key question to be addressed by cytotoxic service managers is whether or not to rotate staff through this service and other departmental activities. A number of factors need to be considered in making such a judgement. The advantages of employing staff specifically to work in the cytotoxic service include assurance that a high level of expertise is established, that speed and efficiency of operations are optimized and such personnel can also fulfil training roles. The disadvantages which require consideration are that the same staff are exposed to the hazards associated with cytotoxic drug handling over long periods, it is more difficult to cover for staff absences and boredom from carrying out the same activities over long periods can lead to lowering of performance.

If a rotational scheme is operated, this ensures that a maximum number of staff are trained and the level of exposure to potentially harmful substances is reduced. However, it is likely that the overall level of competence is lower and more supervision and monitoring may be deemed necessary.

STAFF MONITORING

It is essential to maintain a system of health surveillance for staff directly involved in handling cytotoxics on a routine basis. This may comprise regular general health screening and the use of specific tests to determine if an individual has been exposed to harmful levels of mutagenic substances.

1 Health Surveillance

The cornerstone of an occupational health monitoring process is to give all staff working with cytotoxics a confidential interview, which is designed to review their medical history and offer the opportunity for the staff member to discuss any fears they may have concerning work with such agents. In this way, all new staff are educated about the risks involved which should reinforce information imparted during the training programme. The interview should be repeated at suitable intervals when the employee's exposure record can also be updated. Such interviews are usually recommended on an annual basis.

An exposure record is an essential part of staff surveillance programmes. It should include a record of the amount of time spent, by each staff member, working with cytotoxics, together with a specific record of involvement with accidental spillages or other occurrences which could increase that person's exposure. In addition, all incidents involving accidental exposure, such as gross spillages or needle sticks, must be reported to the Occupational Health department. Blood sampling and a physical examination should be undertaken to identify signs of acute toxicity to skin, mucous membranes, eyes, etc. Records should be maintained centrally, ideally by the Occupational Health or Personnel departments. Computerization of these records allows for rapid data entry and recall, especially if linked to the Pharmacy system used in the operation of the service. Exposure and incident records should be retained with the employee's personal record. A copy should be available on request to any employee who leaves the service or tranfers to another hospital. If a local Occupational Health policy exists, this should be made available to general practitioners, and employees working for an Authority without Occupational Health facilities should be advised to inform their general practitioner of the nature of their work. Many authorities now recommend that staff who are pregnant or contemplating pregnancy should be excluded from duties involving the preparation or administration of cytotoxics.

2 Staff Monitoring for Exposure to Mutagenic Agents

The need to monitor staff for specific biological evidence of enhanced exposure to cytotoxics is controversial. While such a system of staff surveillance offers, in theory, a sensitive means of monitoring the real biological risks to staff, in terms of indices of mutagenicity, test methods currently available do not appear to offer adequate assurance of their ability to identify the real risks. Methods may either be insufficiently sensitive or poorly validated. The following tests are available and, in theory at least, offer a monitoring test for staff. These have recently been assessed by Ferguson et al.[14] All these tests demonstrate statistically significant differences between patients receiving chemotherapy and control groups.

Assay for chromosome aberrations

This method offers the most direct estimate of heritable changes, but is relatively insensitive and laborious to perform. Its main importance lies in the fact that it measures long-lasting lesions and, therefore, provides an index of accumulative /

damage. In fact, if the test indicates that a particular individual does show an increase in chromosomal aberrations with time, this probably indicates that hazardous substances are being absorbed and urgent preventive measures are required.

Micronucleus assay

This method provides a more indirect method of detecting exposure to cytotoxics. The method is less time-consuming to perform than chromosomal aberration tests and does not require the same high level of technical skill, but it is too variable to identify real differences in individuals.[14] However, it may be useful when applied to sufficiently large groups of workers to identify differences between populations or between working conditions. It may be improved by the use of the cytochalasin block method.[15]

Sister chromatid exchange (SCE)

This method detects reciprocal exchanges between chromatids. It is a sensitive method and detects changes that could be caused by very low levels of mutagenic compounds. However, it must be realized that SCE lesions are short-lived and decline substantially within a few days. The test must be performed immediately after the sample has been collected. It will clearly have relevance to testing personnel while working with cytotoxics. It has no retrospective value.

Whether or not routine blood testing of staff for evidence of exposure to mutagenic substances should be conducted remains controversial. Many official guidelines suggest that these tests are not yet sufficiently sensitive nor sufficiently validated to provide meaningful information concerning the levels of risk to which staff have been exposed. However, Ferguson *et al.*[14] argue that a monitoring programme would provide a means of assessing if a relationship may exist between consistent detection of abnormalities and occupational exposure to cytotoxics. Such testing may also provide a warning of equipment failure, poor technique practised by an individual, or inadequacies in protective clothing. The knowledge base relating to staff testing remains insufficient to offer firm guidance on the value or the necessity for such testing.

Ferguson *et al.*[14] suggest that the SCE test is most relevant to testing personnel actively working in cytotoxic services. However, if tests are only performed as a routine on all staff, irrespective of their current duties, the chromosomal aberrations test is the only appropriate method.

CONTROL OF EXPOSURE

1 The Working Environment

All preparation work involving the handling of cytotoxics must be conducted within a suitable safety cabinet or isolator. These are described in Chapter 2. It is also important to appreciate that these facilities require monitoring according to good pharmaceutical practice. Adequate quality control procedures should be established and a testing programme for safety cabinets and isolators should be established and operated by the appropriate quality control staff.

A suitable monitoring programme for a centralized cytotoxic service would normally require the following testing to be performed (*see* BS 5726 and 5295[16,17] for more details):

▼ cabinet complies with KI disc test (determined annually);
▼ airflow direction is inwards over the entire area of the working aperture (for cabinets). Mean flow velocity inwards through the working aperture is 0.4 m/sec (determined quarterly);
▼ airflow velocity of down-flow air complies with BS 5726, ie 0.25–0.50 m/sec (determined quarterly);
▼ manometer readings showing adequate pressure differentials, should be recorded (determined daily).

Microbiological monitoring should also be carried out:

▼ monitor the number of colony-forming units/m^3 of air, using Biotest, air sampler, Sartorius, MD8 sampler or other suitable device (determined quarterly). Limits and action levels should be set;
▼ swab test specified surfaces within each cabinet and Isolator to check microbiological cleanliness (determined quarterly);
▼ agar settle plates in specified areas (determined daily).

Plates should be labelled as having originated from a cytotoxic area. Limits and action levels should be set. Trend analysis would be appropriate in many large units.

2 Handling Precautions

If preparations of cytotoxic work is to be conducted in a safety cabinet, operators must wear appropriate protective clothing (*see* Chapter 3). Extensive training and regular assessment of competence is essential to maintain standards and to ensure staff are protected against the risks associated with handling cytotoxics. Written procedures must be prepared and adhered to by all staff (*see* Chapter 7). It should always be stressed that failure to perform in a safe and competent way by one member of the team will create a potential risk not only for that person but for the other staff working in the Unit. In addition to professional and technical staff, other grades will be involved in handling cytotoxics, eg storekeepers, porters, etc. They need to be educated to an appropriate level in relation to their responsibilities. Furthermore, a procedure for the safe disposal of cytotoxic waste must be available. All those staff involved must be familiar with, and follow established procedures for collecting, segregating and disposing of this waste.

Collection of cytotoxic waste

Suitable containers, clearly labelled and reserved solely for cytotoxic waste, should be available in all areas where the drugs are handled. Glass fragments, needles, etc must be placed in puncture-proof 'Sharps' boxes (*see* Chapter 4), which should be changed on a daily basis. Bulky items require multiple wrapping in plastic bags labelled with the nature of the contents.

Disposal of cytotoxic waste

The disposal of unusual items such as contaminated filters from laminar flow cabinets, is best left to specialist contractors.

A crucial aspect of a waste disposal procedure is the transfer of material from the controlled environment of the Pharmacy working areas to the incinerator or collection point for disposal. If practical, a member of the Pharmacy staff should be delegated to supervise this operation. All staff involved, including Works personnel, must be aware of the procedures. These must be clearly and simply written and must cover all health and safety aspects, including the use of gloves for handling containers and action to be taken in case of breakage.

Segregation and storage of cytotoxics

Since it is necessary to transport cytotoxics around the hospital, a number of factors need to be considered: a method should exist to identify those agents where special precautions are required, eg warning labels on shelves and bins; written procedures for handling damaged packages of cytotoxics should be available; facilities for storage of prepared and waste cytotoxics should be designed to minimize the risks of breakage and methods of transport within the hospital must be chosen to minimize the risk of breakage or leakage.

3 Regulations Controlling Exposure of Staff to Hazardous Substances

Many countries now have statutory controls concerning the protection of staff working with potentially hazardous substances. In the UK, these are primarily covered by the Control of Substances Hazardous to Health (COSHH) Regulations (1988) as part of the Health and Safety at Work Act (1974).[18] The regulations require employers to prevent or control exposure of their employees (or of visitors to their premises) to any substances potentially or actually hazardous to health. Failure of employers to do so can result in criminal prosecution as can failure of employees (or visitors) to comply with any applicable safety procedures or recommendations made by employers. The phrase 'substance hazardous to health' covers almost any type of substance and degree of potential or actual hazard from, for example, concentrated acids through pathogenic micro-organisms to any type of dust. A few substances are specifically excluded because they are covered by existing legislation. Drugs are excluded for the recipient patient but are included if they represent a hazard to health workers handling them. This will include all staff such as nurses and doctors as well as Pharmacy personnel. Cytotoxics are a risk category to be considered.

In summary, the action required of employers by the regulations is to:

▼ identify the substances concerned;
▼ assess the degree of actual risk. This may involve quantitative measurement of exposure levels;
▼ define the safeguards required;
▼ bring these measures to the attention of everyone who needs to know; ensure they are implemented and monitor compliance and effectiveness;
▼ continually monitor the significance of known hazards and respond to the occurrence of potential new ones.

The responsibilities outlined have long been acknowledged by Pharmacists and, in the context of cytotoxics, much work has already been done, for example, the establishment of centralized reconstitution facilities. The regulations do, however, require a more formal approach to this aspect of health and safety than may have been adopted in the past. Proper documentation of policies and procedures is especially important. Pharmacists should be aware that these demands provide added weight to the arguments for establishing a centralized reconstitution and preparation service.

DEALING WITH SPILLAGES

All possible precautions should be taken to avoid accidental spillage.

▼ Adequate training of staff.
▼ Good design of unit and equipment.
▼ Optimal operator protection.
▼ Safe transport of raw materials and finished products.
▼ Safe disposal of waste.

In the event of accidental spillage, personnel should be aware of written procedures for dealing with the problem. These procedures should be drawn up to cover:

▼ spillage within the cytotoxic reconstitution area;
▼ spillage within the wider environs of the Pharmacy department;
▼ spillage within the ward/clinic areas of the hospital. This will involve discussions with nursing, clinical and administrative staff, as well as the hospital's Health and Safety Committee.

1 General Procedure for Dealing with Spillage

▼ Individuals must wear protective clothing which includes double gloves, goggles, plastic apron, etc. (*see* Chapter 3).
▼ Spillages must be contained as far as possible. Dry powder spills should be covered and then the cloth saturated with water.

▼ The spillage should be thoroughly and immediately cleaned up.
▼ Where appropriate, neutralizing solutions should be available, with clear instructions as to their use (*see* individual monographs in Part 2 for details of specific agents).
▼ Adequate quantities of clean water and absorbent paper must be used and disposed of correctly.
▼ Appropriate facilities for the disposal of waste should be available. These include clearly labelled plastic bags of an adequate thickness.
▼ Other staff should be available for assistance if required.

Consideration should be given to the provision of emergency cytotoxic spill-packs, especially for areas remote from the Pharmacy where expert advice may not be available. Emergency spill-packs can be assembled locally, or purchased from a commercial source (eg 'Cytospill', Emergency Cleaning Kit, WM Supplies (UK) Ltd).

2 Cytotoxic Spill-pack

Suggested contents include (*see* also Chapter 3):

▼ protective goggles;
▼ half-face mask;
▼ latex or other similar gloves, 2 pairs (preferably heavy duty);
▼ absorbent towels/gauze pads/granules;
▼ sachets of water for irrigation;
▼ plastic apron;
▼ heavy-gauge plastic bags;
▼ labels, indicating: 'CYTOTOXIC WASTE, for incineration at 1000°C'.

Clear instructions should be included in the pack.

3 Reporting of Spillage Incidents

It is essential that all incidents that involve accidental spillage of cytotoxics are reported as laid down in the procedures document. The report should include the nature of the spillage; where and when it occurred; which staff were directly involved and which staff helped in the cleaning operation; what drugs were involved; approximate quantities and form of the drug and if any direct skin contact or possibilities of absorption occurred.

A full report should be sent to the Occupational Health department, especially if skin absorption etc. may have occurred.

THE DISPOSAL OF CYTOTOXIC DRUGS AND MATERIALS CONTAMINATED WITH THEM

In the UK, prescription-only medicines are listed in Schedule 1 of the *Control of Pollution (Special Waste) Regulations* (1980) as substances which are to be regarded as special waste. There is no specific reference to cytotoxics in these regulations, but their disposal will be subject to the general controls set out therein.

Although the regulations apply to any quantity of 'special waste', however small, there is a need for a commonsense approach to the disposal of unwanted medicines. This has been recognized by the UK Department of the Environment, which gives guidance on the application of the pollution regulations in its joint circular 4/81. The circular recommends householders to dispose of small quantities of unwanted pharmaceuticals by flushing to sewer.[19] Under normal circumstances, the quantity of pharmaceuticals for destruction by an average hospital or Community Pharmacy will be small enough to be disposed of by this method. The disposal of clinical waste is also covered in other UK government publications.[20,21]

The risk associated with pharmaceutical waste which might enter the water cycle has been discussed in detail in a review by Richardson and Bowron.[22] They calculated that the major source of pharmaceutical chemicals as contaminants in potable water would be from domestic sources, including homes and hospitals, with only a marginal contribution to the load from industry. The authors concluded, from analytical and biodegradation data, that few drugs were likely to survive treatment in sewage works, river retention, reservoir retention and waterworks. Such drugs that did survive would be unlikely to pose a health risk at the concentrations likely to be found in water supplies. It can be concluded, therefore, that disposal to sewer may be used for small quantities of pharmaceuticals.

Disposal via the domestic sewerage system should not be used for large quantities of pharmaceutical waste. The Royal Pharmaceutical Society of Great Britain, in their guidelines, recommend Pharmacists to use their professional judgement when deciding on the disposal of substances which may be particularly toxic, insidious or persistent.[23]

The relationship between hazard and the quantities of any particular cytotoxic substance requiring disposal is not generally addressed. However, in the USA, this issue is covered by regulations from the Environmental Protection Agency. These were recently summarized by Gallelli.[24] The relevant 'rules' are described as the '3%' and the 'mixture' rules. The former states that all empty containers that contain not more than 3% of cytotoxics by weight in relation to the total capacity of the container, need not be disposed of as hazardous waste. The 'mixture' rule states that if any amount of a listed waste is mixed with any other, the entire mixture is considered hazardous. This is to prevent the deliberate dilution of cytotoxic waste to avoid disposal regulations.

Many cytotoxics can be disposed of by chemical destruction. Details of recommended methods are summarized in Part 2 of this Handbook. Other important sources of information on chemical destruction of cytotoxics are recommended.[25,26]

A programme of research work is currently being carried out in the UK into methods of visualization of spillages of cytotoxics and into suitable procedures for decontamination and disposal.

Until this work is completed, the method recommended for disposal of cytotoxic drugs is incineration. Disposal into waste which might subsequently be tipped into a landfill site must not, under any circumstances, be used for cytotoxic drugs or materials contaminated with them. Several manufacturers recommend a temperature of 1000°C for the complete destruction of cytotoxic drugs.[27] Opinion differs as to the need for this, but until adequate research work has been carried out, this should be regarded as an ideal to be attained if possible. Perhaps of more importance than the actual temperature is the presence of an after-burner on the incinerator to be used. There is a possible risk of a solution containing a cytotoxic being aerosolized when passed into the incinerator. This may result in undegraded cytotoxic drug being emitted from the incinerator chimney. In the absence of a suitable incinerator, the services of a specialist waste disposal contractor should be employed.

There should be a written policy regarding procedures for the disposal of waste cytotoxics and materials contaminated with them. The procedures must be practicable to operate within the institution. All staff, of whatever grade, who are involved with the handling and disposal of cytotoxics, should be familiar with the details of the policy and procedures. A register should be kept, giving details of the drugs and quantities disposed of by the Pharmacy.

It is essential that there is an arrangement for audit of the policies and procedures laid down, to ensure that there is full compliance at all times with those policies and procedures.

A QUALITY AUDIT SCHEME FOR A CYTOTOXICS RECONSTITUTION SERVICE

The following audit scheme provides a systematic approach to examining the structure and process aspects of a cytotoxic reconstitution service. The main objectives of the audit process are as follows:

▼ To identify shortcomings and loopholes in the procedures and processes.
▼ To determine whether those procedures are being followed and the processes are being carried out effectively by competent staff.
▼ To determine whether the facilities, equipment and environment comply with relevant standards.
▼ To monitor quality trends and assess the effectiveness of management action to remedy perceived deficiencies.
▼ To motivate staff to provide a safe, efficient and cost-effective service.

The audit form (Table 6.1) incorporates a rating scale for level of compliance and also guidance on the means of assessment for each acceptance criterion. For some criteria, the assessment depends upon a process of peer review and it is, therefore, important that auditors have appropriate expertise.

This audit scheme is not proffered as a definitive statement applicable to all situations; it is intended to be a model which can be adapted to local circumstances. It should also be regarded as one of a number of quality assurance mechanisms that can be applied. It does not, for instance, attempt to address the outcomes of the patient's treatment.

1 Notes for Guidance when using Quality Audit Forms

Result ratings

1. Substantial compliance with Acceptance Criteria.
2. Significant compliance with Acceptance Criteria.
3. Partial compliance with Acceptance Criteria.
4. Minimal compliance with Acceptance Criteria.
5. Noncompliance with Acceptance Criteria.

NA Not applicable

Glossary of terms used in connection with the checks required for each criterion.

Assess	requires the auditor(s) to use their professional judgement in attributing a compliance rating.
Data	generally relates to validation studies and evidence taken from the literature.
Examine	generally relates to procedures and/or materials which need to be examined, for content and validity.
Observe	generally relates to activities which can be observed by auditor(s) and are representative of normal work practices. In some situations it may be appropriate to do this covertly.
Procedure	relates to written procedures which should be assessed for appropriateness and compliance with official guidelines (eg good manufacturing practice). They should have been recently appraised, signed and, where appropriate, countersigned (eg by Quality Control staff).
Records	generally relates to requirements for documentary evidence. These should be inspected at the auditor(s) discretion.
Test	applies to situations where the auditor(s) obtain their own evidence by test.

Table 6.1: *Quality audit for cytotoxic reconstitutions*

HOSPITAL:	DATE:	CYTOTOXIC REGIMEN EXAMINED:			BATCH NO(S):
No.	Attribute	Acceptance Criteria	Check Req'd	Audit Result	Comments and Action to be Taken
001	Formulation acceptability	All formulations are stable (published or in-house evidence)	Data	1 2 3 4 5 NA	
002		All formulations are approved (with signature) by a Pharmacist	Examine	1 2 3 4 5 NA	
003		Dose is for a single patient's requirements only	Procedure	1 2 3 4 5 NA	
005	Facilities	Facilities are adequate size for the activities undertaken	Assess	1 2 3 4 5 NA	
006		Facilities incorporate appropriate design features in terms of current GMP, ergonomics, work flow, ease of cleaning etc	Assess	1 2 3 4 5 NA	
007		Facilities include sufficient shelves, cupboards, benches etc for the activities undertaken	Assess	1 2 3 4 5 NA	
008		Walls, floors, ceilings, fixtures and fittings have acceptable finish and in good decorative order	Assess	1 2 3 4 5 NA	
	Environmental acceptability product protection	(A) Applicable to use of modified Class 2 (BS 5726) Microbiological Safety Cabinet			
009		Room used complies with (at least) Class J (unmanned) air (BS 5295) and tested within 3 months	Records	1 2 3 4 5 NA	
010		Safety cabinet complies with Class E (manned) air (BS 5295) and tested within 3 months	Records	1 2 3 4 5 NA	
011		The direction of the air-flow is inwards over the whole area of the work aperture (Smoke test confirmation)	Records/Test	1 2 3 4 5 NA	
012		The velocity of the down-flow air is in accordance with the requirements of BS 5726 (0.25–0.5 m/sec)	Records	1 2 3 4 5 NA	
013		The mean air velocity through the working aperture by measurement of the exhaust velocity meets the requirements of BS 5726	Records	1 2 3 4 5 NA	
014		Safety cabinet and room comply with in-house standard for absence of micro-organisms and tested within one week	Records	1 2 3 4 5 NA	

Table 6.1: *continued*

No.	Attribute	Acceptance Criteria	Check Req'd	Audit Result	Comments and Action to be Taken
015		Cleanroom garments/face mask/gloves used each session (see also 020)	Observe/ Procedure	1 2 3 4 5 NA	
016		Cleaning records comply with schedule	Records	1 2 3 4 5 NA	
017		Manometer readings show adequate differential pressure (if appropriate) and are recorded daily	Records	1 2 3 4 5 NA	
	Environmental acceptability product protection	(B) Applicable to use of negative pressure isolator system			
018		Air complies with Class E (manned) air (BS 5295) within 2 minutes of opening and closing the transfer hatch and tested within 3 months	Records	1 2 3 4 5 NA	
019		Environment complies with in-house standard for absence of micro-organisms and tested within one week	Records	1 2 3 4 5 NA	
020		Cleaning records comply with schedule including fumigation of inside of cabinet when applicable	Records	1 2 3 4 5 NA	
021		The cabinet alarm system operates if the cabinet's seals are breached	Assess	1 2 3 4 5 NA	
022	Environment acceptability operator protection	Safety cabinet complies with KI Discus test and tested within one year (not applicable for isolators)	Records	1 2 3 4 5 NA	
023		Systems prevent disturbance of air currents during use of cabinet, including opening/closing of door to room (not applicable for isolators)	Procedure/ Assess	1 2 3 4 5 NA	
024		Appropriate type of garments including gloves used by staff	Assess	1 2 3 4 5 NA	
025		The glove/sleeve system allows adequate dexterity in use and gloves are replaced as necessary (isolators only)	Assess	1 2 3 4 5 NA	
026		Luer-lock syringes and large-bore needles used during manipulations	Observe/ Procedure	1 2 3 4 5 NA	
027		Appropriate air-venting of vials occurs to prevent pressure differentials	Observe/ Procedure	1 2 3 4 5 NA	
028		Acceptable procedure for dealing with spillage in existence	Examine	1 2 3 4 5 NA	

Table 6.1: *continued*

No.	Attribute	Acceptance Criteria	Check Req'd	Audit Result	Comments and Action to be Taken
029		Appropriate receptacles for contaminated liquids, 'sharps' and other consumables available	Assess	1 2 3 4 5 NA	
030		Appropriate procedure for disposal of contaminated waste available	Examine	1 2 3 4 5 NA	
031	Documentation (General)	Satisfactory standard operating procedures have been written for all items of equipment and signed and dated by the production Pharmacist and independent quality control Pharmacist	Examine	1 2 3 4 5 NA	
032		Worksheets for all different cytotoxic preparations have been written and signed and dated by the Pharmacist and independent quality control Pharmacist	Examine	1 2 3 4 5 NA	
033		Satisfactory procedures have been written, signed and dated on the following:			
		i) Changing and hand-washing prior to entry into preparation area (and is displayed)	Examine/ Observe	1 2 3 4 5 NA	
		ii) Laboratory cleaning and maintenance	Examine	1 2 3 4 5 NA	
		iii) Environmental and microbiological control	Examine	1 2 3 4 5 NA	
		iv) Other routine quality control testing	Examine	1 2 3 4 5 NA	
		v) Health and Safety policy	Examine	1 2 3 4 5 NA	
034	Compounding	Documentary evidence of correct reconstitution	Records	1 2 3 4 5 NA	
035		Other documentary evidence completed and satisfactory	Records	1 2 3 4 5 NA	
036		Evidence to show that correct solutions incorporated into syringe/bag	Observe	1 2 3 4 5 NA	
037		Appropriate sterile filters used	Observe/ Procedure	1 2 3 4 5 NA	
038	Presentation	Label has acceptable legibility	Examine Sample	1 2 3 4 5 NA	
039		Label bears unambiguous expression of ingredients/quantities	Examine Sample	1 2 3 4 5 NA	
040		Label shows correct expiry date/time	Examine Sample	1 2 3 4 5 NA	
041		Label shows correct storage conditions if other than room temperature	Examine Sample	1 2 3 4 5 NA	

Table 6.1: *continued*

No.	Attribute	Acceptance Criteria	Check Req'd	Audit Result	Comments and Action to be Taken
042		Outer packaging is properly sealed and prevents contents leaking during transit	Examine Sample	1 2 3 4 5 NA	
043		Contents clear and practically free from visible particles	Examine Sample	1 2 3 4 5 NA	
044	Personnel	Appropriately trained and screened Pharmacists/Pharmacy technicians undertake the manipulations	Assess	1 2 3 4 5 NA	
045		All personnel are aware of and comply with the local policy on handling of cytotoxic materials	Assess	1 2 3 4 5 NA	
046		Staff perform satisfactory broth transfers every 6 months	Records	1 2 3 4 5 NA	
047	Effective use of resources	Notification of Pharmacy by ward allows convenient scheduling	Assess	1 2 3 4 5 NA	
048		Most cost effective grade(s) of staff are used	Assess	1 2 3 4 5 NA	
049		Choice of units of ingredients minimizes wastage	Assess	1 2 3 4 5 NA	
050		The ingredients bear the nearest expiry date of stock	Examine	1 2 3 4 5 NA	
051		The wastage of disposables used is minimal	Observe	1 2 3 4 5 NA	
052	Storage/distribution and administration	Contents are suitably protected against heat/light etc	Examine	1 2 3 4 5 NA	
053		Syringes/bags are suitably protected for transport to ward	Examine	1 2 3 4 5 NA	
054		Bags can be delivered to ward by intended time of administration	Assess	1 2 3 4 5 NA	
055		Syringes/bags are appropriately stored on the ward if not to be used immediately and do not exceed their expiry date	Assess	1 2 3 4 5 NA	

	NAME:	JOB TITLE:	SIGNATURE:	DATE:
Auditor 1:				
Auditor 2:				
Auditor 3:				
Other staff present:				
Copies sent to:				
Next Audit date:				

REFERENCES

1. Sieber, S.M. and Adamson, R.H. (1975). Toxicity of antineoplastic agents in man: chromosomal aberrations, antifertility effects, congenital malformations and carcinogenic potential. *Adv. Cancer Res.* **22**, 57–155.
2. Boice, J.D. *et al.* (1983). Leukemia and preleukemia after adjuvent treatment of gastrointestinal cancer with semustine (methyl-CCNU). *New Eng. J. Med.* **309**, 1079–1084.
3. Selevan, S.G. *et al.* (1985). A study of occupational exposure to antineoplastic drugs and fetal loss in nurses. *New Eng. J. Med.* **313**, 1173–1178.
4. Hemminki, K. *et al.* (1985). Spontaneous abortions and malformations in the offspring of nurses exposed to anaesthetic gases, cytotoxic drugs and other potential hazards in hospitals, based on registered information of outcome. *J. Epid. and Comm. Health*, **39**, 141–147.
5. Falck, K. (1982). *Application of the bacterial urinary mutagenicity assay in detection of exposure to genotoxic chemicals.* PhD dissertation, University of Helisinki, pp. 55.
6. Andersson, R.W. *et al.* (1982). Risks of handling injectable antineoplastic drugs. *Am. J. Hosp. Pharm.* **39**, 1881–1887.
7. Falck, K. *et al.* (1979). Mutagencity in urine of nurses handling cytotoxic drugs. *Lancet*, **1**, 1250–1251.
8. Norppa, H. *et al.* (1980). Increased sister chromatid exchange frequencies in lymphocytes of nurses handling cytotoxic drugs. *Scand. J. Work and Environ. Health*, **6**, 299–303.
9. Sorsa, M. *et al.* (1982). Induction of sister chromatid exchanges (SCE's) among nurses handling cytotoxic drugs. *Banbury Proc.* Vol. 14. Cold Spring Harbor Laboratory, New York.
10. Waksvik, H. *et al.* (1981). Chromosome analyses of nurses handling cytotoxic drugs. *Cancer Treat. Rep.* **65**, 607–611.
11. Vainio, H. (1982). Mutagenicity in urine of workers occupationally exposed to mutagens and carcinogens. In Aito, A. *et al.* (Eds): *Biological monitoring and health surveillance of workers exposed to chemicals.* Hemisphere Publishing, Washington DC, 324–330.
12. Cooke, J. (1987). Environmental monitoring of personnel who handle cytotoxic drugs. *Pharm. J.* **239**, R2.
13. Kolmodin-Hedman, B. *et al.* (1983). Occupational handling of cytotoxic drugs. *Arch. Tox.* **54**, 25–33.
14. Ferguson, L.R. *et al.* (1988). The use within New Zealand of cytogenetic approaches to monitoring of hospital pharmacists for exposure to cytotoxic drugs: report of a pilot study in Auckland. *Aust. J. of Hosp. Pharm.* **18**, 228–233.
15. Fenech, M. *et al.* (1986). Cytokinesis-block micronucleus method in human lymophocytes: effect of *in vivo* aging and low-dose X-irradiation. *Mutation Res.* **161**, 193–198.
16. Anon. (1979). *Specification for microbiological safety cabinets, BS 5726.* British Standards Institute, London.

17. Anon. (1989). *Environmental cleanliness in enclosed spaces, Parts 1, 2, 3, BS 5295*. British Standards Institute, London.
18. Anon. (1988). *The control of substances hazardous to health regulations*. HMSO, London.
19. Anon. (1980). *Joint circular from Department of Environment/Welsh Office, Control of Pollution (Special Waste) regulations*. HMSO, London.
20. Anon. (1983). *Department of Environment waste paper No. 25, chemical wastes*. HMSO, London.
21. Anon. (1982). *The safe disposal of chemical waste*, Health and Safety Commission. HMSO, London.
22. Richardson, M.L. and Bowron, G.M. (1985). The fate of pharmaceutical chemicals in the aquatic environment. *J. Pharm. Pharmac.* **37**, 1–12.
23. Appleby, G.E. (1988). Disposal of pharmaceutical waste. *Pharm. J.* **240**, 100.
24. Gallelli, J.F. (1988). Chemical destruction and disposal of antineoplastic drugs. In: *Proceedings of international symposium on oncology pharmacy practice, Rotorua, New Zealand*. New Zealand Hospital Pharmacists Association, Wellington, pp. 240–251.
25. Castegnaro, M. *et al.* (1985). *Laboratory decontamination and destruction of carcinogens in laboratory wastes*: International Agency for Research on Cancer, Scientific Publications No. 73, Oxford University Press, Fair Lane (N.J.).
26. Armour, M.A. *et al.* (1986). *Potentially carcinogenic chemicals: information and disposal guide*, University of Alberta. Terochem Laboratories Ltd, Edmonton.
27. Garner, S. *et al.* (1988). Disposal of waste cytotoxics. *Pharm. J.* **241**, Hospital Supplement 32.

CHAPTER 7

Documentation

INTRODUCTION

Adequate and efficient documentation is an essential aspect of a Pharmacy-operated cytotoxic service. The design of documentation is clearly of importance in ensuring the maintenance of safe procedures and good records of service operation. The range of documents used, their design, reproduction and updating aspects will vary widely between hospitals. They will be governed by local circumstances such as the scale of operation, the grades of staff involved and the extent to which computers are used.

It may be considered that for some services, documents can be combined or contain superfluous information. However, in this text all those aspects that require consideration have been indicated. Local circumstances then dictate whether or not they are included in the user documentation.

Whether the storage and retrieval system devised is computerized or not, the basic needs of documentation remain the same.

DOCUMENTATION NEEDS

The various aspects of cytotoxics services requiring documents for safe, reliable and cost-effective operation are shown in Figure 7.1. The actual document needs have been summarized under each of the main categories depicted in the figure.

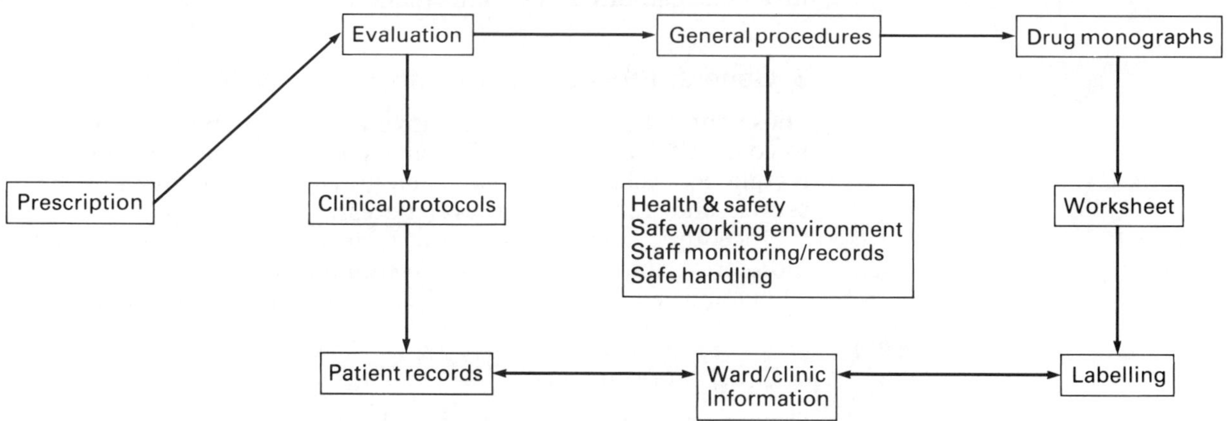

Figure 7.1: *Documentation required for cytotoxic services*

1 Prescriptions

There are several options regarding the ordering of chemotherapy.

▼ The patient's prescription may be sent to the Pharmacy department.
▼ The patient's prescription may be transposed at ward or clinic level by the visiting Pharmacist.
▼ A specially designed order form completed by the clinician may be supplied to the Pharmacy. This may have a worksheet incorporated in its design.
▼ Visual display units or fax machines may be used with terminals at ward, clinic and Pharmacy level.

2 Clinical Protocols

Chemotherapy regimens are divided mainly into two groups.

▼ Protocols that are part of a formal clinical trial.
▼ Regimens which are based on experience and subject to the clinician's expertise and judgement, many of them being standard first-line treatments.

Clinical trial protocols are often complex and subject to randomization. For quick reference it may be appropriate to summarize the pharmaceutical aspects in a card or file system which details:

▼ schedules (induction, consolidation, maintenance, etc.)
▼ drug
▼ dose ($/m^2$ or $/kg$)
▼ how given (route, volume, equipment)
▼ timings (pulses, cycles, etc.)
▼ dosage reductions (when and how appropriate).

For standard treatment regimens, compilations of similar data from reference or from clinical sources can also be prepared. However, these are more likely to need updating frequently and hospital Drug Information units may be the appropriate means of gathering such information.

3 General Procedures (*see* also Chapter 6)

These should be clear, informative and comprehensive enough to cover all aspects of the Pharmacy service. They should be readily accessible, comprehensible to all staff employed in the service and updated whenever necessary.

  Procedures covering personnel; education and training; staff monitoring; handling (suitable techniques and methods of evaluation) and waste disposal are of particular importance.

4 Drug Monographs

Drug monographs for commercially available injectable cytotoxic drugs are contained in part 2 of this Handbook.

5 Worksheets

A general worksheet may be used for all drugs or specific worksheets may be prepared for particular regimens. Prescription details can be transcribed on to the worksheet or the worksheet can be an integral part of the prescription.
  Worksheets should include:

▼ name of the drug/s
▼ presentation (physical form, quantity, strength, etc.)
▼ reconstituting solutions/diluents (identification and quantities to be added)
▼ resultant solutions (quantity in volume)
▼ compatible infusion solutions (where appropriate)
▼ storage details
▼ stability
▼ labelling details or sample label
▼ pertinent 'special precautions' (eg carmustine vials should be inspected before use for signs of decomposition of the drug).

They should allow the following to be recorded:

▼ batch numbers of all ingredients used
▼ the number of containers used
▼ the quantities of solutions to be drawn up or removed
▼ label duplicate
▼ identification of personnel involved in the preparation stages (formulation, assembly of ingredients, reconstitution, etc.)
▼ identification of personnel involved in the checking procedures.

6 Labelling

Labels should comply with national regulations and should state the:

▼ intended route of administration
▼ name of the drug
▼ quantity of the drug
▼ vehicle containing the drug (infusion solution as appropriate)
▼ final volume
▼ batch number allocated to the product
▼ expiry date
▼ storage conditions that ensure stability, etc.
▼ patient's name and location (ward, etc.)
▼ name and address of the cytotoxic dispensary.

Outer packs for transport should also clearly state details of the contained items and any possible handling hazards.

7 Information Documents for Ward/Clinic Staff

These should comprise the elements listed below. The detail required will depend on local circumstance.

General introduction detailing local policies

These may include:

▼ designated areas on ward/clinic for the preparation of cytotoxic agents
▼ personnel (ie groups of staff appropriate to undertake reconstitution/administration)
▼ protective garments that should be worn
▼ equipment that may be used
▼ extravasation policies
▼ disposal of waste.

Drug monographs

These will obviously be much less detailed than those required in Pharmacy.

▼ presentation
▼ reconstitution
▼ compatible solutions
▼ methods of administration
▼ special precautions (operator safety, extravasation, etc.)
▼ stability
▼ accidental spillage (what to do in the event of).

Arrangements for the supply of cytotoxics from the Pharmacy

▼ procedure for the agreed method of service-operation at ward level (eg how and when to order)
▼ communication access (personnel to contact, telephone numbers, etc.)
▼ agreed presentations and possible alternatives for each drug.

8 Patient Records

These can comprise any relevant information that the Pharmacy service requires for its specific needs. Records kept on computer are subject to the Data Protection Act in the UK.

To ensure a comprehensive and efficient checking process the following information should be available:

▼ patient's name
▼ address or hospital number
▼ date of birth
▼ diagnosis
▼ protocol/drug regimen
▼ surface area
▼ consultant.

In addition, a Pharmacy history can be compiled to include:

▼ chemotherapy supplied to the patient to date
▼ dates of when chemotherapy given (can assist in predicting when the patient is next expected to receive further treatment)
▼ anomalies (dosage reductions, missed pulses, fluid restriction, etc.)
▼ changes in regimens, relapse, etc.

COMPUTER TECHNOLOGY

Computer technology has an important role to play in three areas of the operation of a cytotoxic reconstitution service; namely labelling and documentation, patient therapy profiling and data management.

The facility to produce (and replicate) detailed, accurate, informative and legible labels to a predetermined and well-designed format is essential. In addition, the speedy reproduction of worksheets and prescriptions and the ability to store and update them easily is fundamental to the success of a busy service.

Computer-based patient chemotherapy profiles are an invaluable aid to safe operation of a high quality service. The data held becomes the first point of reference for both technical and clinical queries and may also form the basis of a detailed and accurate costing system.

A 'traditional' dispensing and stock control facility allows collection, collation and easy retrieval of data on the operation of the service and can be a valuable management tool, allowing monitoring and measurement of performance, service levels and drug use efficiency.

The choice of computer system depends largely on the individual user, operational requirements, pre-existing computer hardware and software and cost. Many centres have designed systems to suit their needs and a number of commercially available software packages can be adapted to suit individual needs.

Education and Training

INTRODUCTION

All staff employed to handle cytotoxic materials should receive education and training appropriate to their level of involvement in the handling, preparation or administration of the drugs.

A training programme should include practical experience, one-to-one teaching, learning exercises which may be tested and information on Health and Safety. A more advanced programme will also include clinical and theoretical training.

The check-list on page 71–3 can be used as the starting point for a formal training programe. Particular sections of the check-list are discussed in more detail below.

PRACTICAL TRAINING

Practical experience in basic aseptic technique is essential before staff are involved in cytotoxic manipulation.

Staff who reconstitute cytotoxics should understand the theory behind the use of these agents in the treatment of cancer and why they are hazardous to handle. Reconstitution techniques should be taught and assessed using non-hazardous materials until the operative's technique has been validated. Standard tests which can be used to simulate in-use situations include:

▼ the aseptic transfer of 1% w/v quinine hydrochloride solution. This fluoresces under UV light indicating spills and poor cleaning technique;
▼ the transfer of liquids between pressurized vials containing water coloured with amaranth or methylene blue dye is useful to demonstrate and eliminate aerosol formation.

The use of all equipment should be demonstrated and backed up by written procedures. All staff should be familiar with written documentation; how to record and calculate doses; labelling and packaging systems. The rationale behind expiry dates and storage conditions should be explained.

THEORY

Both formal and informal schemes may be operated for all grades of staff, appropriate to their level of responsibility.

Formal schemes involve detailed procedure notes, drug information, recommended texts and attendance at lectures and study days. Provision for continuing education and monitoring of validated staff is often overlooked but is essential for quality assurance of the service.

Senior staff should be expected to participate in the planning and development of the service.

CLINICAL TRAINING

The degree of clinical involvement varies between units and even individual Pharmacists in the same unit. It is essential to retain first-hand clinical contact wherever practicable.

Staff involved in the clinical setting should undertake a formal clinical training programme in addition to the practical training programme. Such a programme should include: one-to-one teaching of oncology/haematology in the clinical setting, by a member of the oncology team; the preparation of case presentations and patient profiles; pharmacokinetic interpretation of dosage schedules; evaluation of new equipment and techniques and involvement in clinical trials and practice research.

THE TRAINING CHECK-LIST

This can be used as the starting point for a formal or informal training programme. Staff may use the list simply as a guide to the areas which should be covered, or a more extensive programme may be written around the headings in the check-list.

The aim of the check-list (*see* Table 8.1) is that staff acquire knowledge of and competence in aseptic procedures, cytotoxic reconstitution, local procedures, current awareness, active information, management and research and development. These are intended as broad guidelines for training. Local variations will exist depending upon circumstance.

The degree of training required in each section depends on the level of involvement of different groups of staff in the provision of chemotherapy. The staff groups are indicated at the top of each column.

Level 1 Full time and rotational technicians involved with the provision of a cytotoxic reconstitution service.

Level 2 Pre-registration Pharmacists, basic grade Pharmacists and senior Pharmacists from other specialities.

Level 3 Senior Pharmacists and technical staff managing a sterile preparation or cytotoxic reconstitution service.

Level 4 District or Regional cytotoxic/oncology Pharmacists.

Training for staff at levels 1 and 2 may be undertaken by staff at levels 3 or 4; at level 3 by those at level 4 and at level 4 by peer review, self-development training courses and engagement of outside expertise.

Where the time available is limited (ie rotational staff), priority should be given to training in aseptic procedures, cytotoxic reconstitution and local procedures. It is anticipated that this should take at least four weeks in a well-resourced unit. However, basic awareness of the relevant techniques can be achieved in two weeks.

Table 8.1: *Education and training check-list*

	Full time and rotational technicians involved with the provision of a cytotoxic reconstitution service	Pre-reg Pharmacists, basic grade Pharmacists and senior Pharmacists from other specialities	Senior Pharmacists and technical staff managing a sterile preparation or cytotoxic reconstitution service	District or Regional cytotoxic oncology Pharmacists
ASEPTIC TECHNIQUE				
What it is	A	A	A	A
Why it is needed	A	A	A	A
How is it achieved	A	A	A	A
Test for ensuring and maintaining it	A	A	A	A
How to realize it has failed	A	A	A	A
What to do when it fails	A	A	A	A
CYTOTOXIC RECONSTITUTION				
What are cytotoxics	A	A	A	A
Why are they a hazard	A	A	A	A
How aerosols are generated	A	A	A	A
How aerosols are prevented	A	A	A	A
Other possible routes of exposure/contamination	A	A	A	A
General reconstitution techniques	A	A	A	A
Special reconstitution techniques	A	A	A	A
Use of special equipment	A	A	A	A
Correct documentation	A	A	A	A
Expiry + storage	A	A	A	A
Tests for ensuring and maintaining good technique	A	A	A	A
LOCAL PROCEDURES				
For aseptic technique	A	A	A	A
For cytotoxic reconstitution	A	A	A	A
USE OF EQUIPMENT				
Special reconstitution devices	A	A	A	A
Special administration devices	I	I	I	I
Evaluation of new equipment	A	A	A	A

Key: A (activity) – denotes activities which trainees would be expected to perform routinely
I (information) – denotes activities which trainees should either be aware of, or engage in less frequently

Table 8.1: *continued*

	Full time and rotational technicians involved with the provision of a cytotoxic reconstitution service	Pre-reg Pharmacists, basic grade Pharmacists and senior Pharmacists from other specialities	Senior Pharmacists and technical staff managing a sterile preparation or cytotoxic reconstitution service	District or Regional cytotoxic oncology Pharmacists
CLINICAL DATA/PHARMACEUTICAL DATA				
Clinical notes	I	A	A	A
Laboratory tests	I	A	A	A
Disease evaluation tests	I	I	A	A
Clinical/nursing procedures	I	I	A	A
Administration procedures	A	A	A	A
Practical pharmacokinetics	I	A	A	A
EVALUATION OF INFORMATION				
Publications	I	A	A	A
Protocols	I	I	A	A
Basic statistics	A	A	A	A
Drug representatives	A	A	A	A
Promotional material	I	I	A	A
Spoken communications	A	A	A	A
OBTAINING DRUG/CLINICAL INFORMATION				
In-house	A	A	A	A
Reading list	I	A	A	A
Library	I	A	A	A
Oral communications	A	A	A	A
On-line via Drug Information Centre	I	I	A	A
DATA HANDLING				
Protocols	A	A	A	A
Documentation	A	A	A	A
Work-load statistics	I	I	A	A
Records	I	I	A	A
Clinical data	I	I	A	A
Adverse reaction reporting	I	I	A	A
Extravasation procedure	I	A	A	A
Mechanism of action	I	A	A	A
Overdose	I	A	A	A
Interactions with other drugs	I	A	A	A
Kinetics	I	I	A	A
Disposal	A	A	A	A
Legal and ethical considerations	I	A	A	A
HEALTH AND SAFETY REGULATIONS				
Nationally	I	I	A	A
Locally	A	A	A	A
Staff screening	I	I	I	A
Accident reporting	A	A	A	A
Accident procedure	A	A	A	A

Key: A (activity)   – denotes activities which trainees would be expected to perform routinely
     I (information) – denotes activities which trainees should either be aware of, or engage in less frequently

Table 8.1: *continued*

	Full time and rotational technicians involved with the provision of a cytotoxic reconstitution service	Pre-reg Pharmacists, basic grade Pharmacists and senior Pharmacists from other specialities	Senior Pharmacists and technical staff managing a sterile preparation or cytotoxic reconstitution service	District or Regional cytotoxic oncology Pharmacists
HEALTH SERVICE BACKGROUND				
NHS framework for the provision of cytotoxic services	I	I	I	I
Current awareness	A	A	A	A
ACTIVE INFORMATION				
Bulletins	I	I	A	A
Seminars	I	I	A	A
Lectures	I	I	A	A
MANAGEMENT				
Education/training of appropriate pharmaceutical, nursing and medical staff	–	–	A	A
Monitoring of service quality	–	I	A	A
Work planning	A	A	A	A
Committee skills	–	–	I	A
Finance/budgeting	–	–	A	A
Interviewing	–	–	A	A
Guidelines for protocol submission preparation and evaluation	–	–	I	A
RESEARCH AND DEVELOPMENT				
Service development	–	–	A	A
Technique evaluation	–	–	A	A
Drug evaluation	–	–	A	A
Publication	–	–	A	A

Key: A (activity)   – denotes activities which trainees would be expected to perform routinely
      I (information) – denotes activities which trainees should either be aware of, or engage in less frequently

CHAPTER 9

Extravasation

INTRODUCTION

Many cytotoxic agents have an irritant, vesicant or allergenic action and can cause local damage to skin and mucous membranes. Extravasation, injection into the extra vascular tissue, due to poor positioning of a needle in a vein, or the 'corrosive' action of certain drugs can lead to severe inflammation and necrosis which, if left untreated, may cause permanent damage requiring plastic surgery.

A better understanding of the hazards of these drugs, increased expertise in methods of administration and advances in the equipment available for administration (Chapters 5 and 10) have helped to minimize the occurrence of extravasation episodes. However, there is still a need for clear guidelines on how to deal with an episode if it occurs.

There are various published articles on anecdotal treatments for extravasation of cytotoxics as well as recommendations from manufacturers.[1–7] However, there is little controlled, clinical evidence to substantiate the efficacy of the treatments. In some cases the recommended antidote would cause further tissue damage in its own right if not used with extreme care (for example, sodium bicarbonate injection) and controversy still surrounds the decision between hot or cold applications. Information on the possible toxicity of the cytotoxic and specific antidotes, if available, are included in the drug monographs later in this handbook.

The information on drugs associated with severe necrosis given in McNeece and Lighty[4] is being extensively updated and should be used for guidance only. However, drugs that are associated with severe local necrosis include dactinomycin, daunorubicin, doxorubicin, epirubicin, etoposide, mithramycin, mitomycin, mustine, vinblastine, vincristine and vindesine.

RECOGNITION OF CYTOTOXIC EXTRAVASATION

Extravasation should be suspected if one or more of the following is observed.

▼ The patient complains of burning, stinging pain or any other acute change at the injection site. This should be distinguished from a feeling of cold which may occur with some drugs.
▼ Induration or swelling at the injection site is observed. There may be redness or 'blistering' with doxorubicin and other red drugs (the 'nettle rash' effect) which is normal.

▼ No blood is obtained. If found in isolation this should not be regarded as an indication of a non-patent vein.
▼ A resistance is felt on the plunger of the syringe if drugs are given by bolus injection.
▼ There is absence of free flow when administration is by infusion.

TREATMENT OF EXTRAVASATION

Every centre preparing or administering cytotoxics should have a local policy for the treatment of extravasation of cytotoxic drugs. The policy should give guidance on the first line treatment of extravasation and meaures to be taken following initial therapy. The policy should include:

▼ general measures to be taken once extravasation has been identified
▼ details of those cytotoxics most likely to cause tissue damage
▼ information on specific antidotes, if known
▼ details of records to be kept
▼ further action.

Each preparation and treatment area should also be supplied with an extravasation kit, containing all the necessary drugs and equipmment to deal with an emergency situation.

The following information, taken from The Royal Marsden Hospital, *Manual of clinical nursing procedures*, 1988,[8] gives an example of general emergency policy for dealing with cytotoxic extravasation details of the type of documentation required and an example of an extravasation treatment kit.

1 General Measures to Take Once Extravasation Has Been Recognized

▼ Stop the injection immediately, leaving the needle in place.
▼ Withdraw 3–5 ml of blood to remove as much of the drug as possible from the site of injection.
▼ Remove the infusion needle so that the site can no longer be used as an intravenous route.
▼ Apply ice or a cold pack.
▼ Draw up dexamethasone injection, 8 mg and inject, subcutaneously volumes of 0.1 to 0.2 ml at the points of the compass around the circumference of the area of extravasation.
▼ Where possible elevate the extremity to minimize swelling and/or encourage movement.
▼ Re-apply ice or cold pack for 15 minutes four times a day.
▼ Apply 1% hydrocortisone cream, twice daily as long as erythema persists.
▼ Observe region for pain, erythema, induration/necrosis.
▼ If ulcerated, seek surgical advice – early excision may be advisable if area is large or persistently painful, as drugs may persist in tissues and continue to cause damage.

▼ If not ulcerated, advise gradual return to normal use of arm, but review regularly and consider surgical excision if persistent pain, swelling or delayed ulceration occur.

2 Documentation (*see* Figure 9.1)

The document should detail:

▼ date, time
▼ needle size
▼ type
▼ location
▼ drug sequence
▼ drug administration technique
▼ approximate amount of extravasated drug
▼ diameter of erythematous area
▼ appearance
▼ patients' complaints and statements
▼ nursing management
▼ nurse's signature.

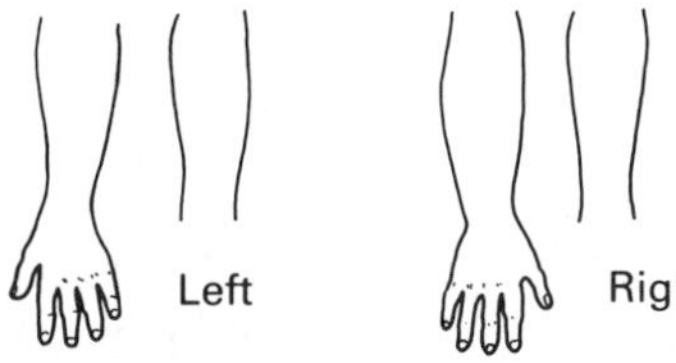

Explain to the patient that the site may remain sore for several days.

In-patients should be monitored daily. Out-patients should be asked to observe the site daily and immediately report any increased discomfort or significant change, such as peeling or blistering of the skin. All information should be recorded.

Figure 9.1: *Extravasation documentation slip*

IN CONFIDENCE REGISTER OF EXTRAVASATION AND ITS TREATMENT

Patient   Male*/Female*   Age ....   Height (m) ....   Weight (kg) ....

Drug causing extravasation was   ....   Dose ....

Infused in* ....   Added to last running drip of * ....   / Stat*

Given Cannula/Butterfly (please state size) ....over .... mins/hr

The above drug formed part of course No. .... in the following regimen

Drug	Total Dose	Infusion Fluid/Stat	Time	Already Given	Not Yet Given
				Yes/No*	Yes/No*
				Yes/No*	Yes/No*
				Yes/No*	Yes/No*
				Yes/No*	Yes/No*

Other drugs being given concurrently (oral + IV's)

Please indicate SITE and canulation and area of extravasation with measurements on the diagrams below

Front   Back   Left or Right Arm*

Other area (please specify) ....

Details of extravasation treatment (Drug, Dose, Procedure) ....

____

____

____

____

Date of extravasation ....   Time ....

Extravasation treatment Started on .... Stopped on .... Outcome ....

This section is not compulsory
Contact name for further details (Dr, nurse, pharmacist) Name .... Tel No ....

Date .... New report*/Follow up*

Additional comments ____

____

____

____

____

* Please delete or fill in as appropriate

____

Figure 9.2: *Example of a 'Green Card'*

3 Contents of an Extravasation Treatment Kit

▼ Injection, dexamethasone 8 mg in 2 ml × 1.
▼ Cream, hydrocortisone 1% 15 g × 1.
▼ Syringes, 2 ml × 2.
▼ Needles, 25 g × 2.
▼ Extravasation management – procedure.
▼ Documentation slip
▼ Spirit swabs.
▼ Instant cold pack.

REPORTING OF EXTRAVASATION EPISODES

In an attempt to collate and analyse data on extravasation events in a large number of patients, a 'Green Card' scheme for reporting extravasation incidences, their treatment and outcome is being co-ordinated through the St Chads Unit, Dudley Road Hospital, Birmingham, UK.

The aim of the scheme is to obtain accurate statistics on the number of extravasation incidents occurring, the drugs involved and the type of therapy being used; to collect data on treatment methods and antidotes used for extravasation incidents; to obtain accurate information on the outcome of the incidents; to feed-back information on treatments and their effectiveness to the clinicians and to produce standard guidelines for the treatment of extravasation.

The reporting cards are available from hospital Pharmacy departments or Oncology units in the UK or can be obtained direct from the Extravasation Report Co-ordinator,
c/o St Chads Unit, Dudley Road Hospital, Birmingham
B18 7QH, UK.

An example of the 'Green Card' is shown in Figure 9.2.

REFERENCES

1. Dorr, R.T. (1981). Extravasation of vessicant antineoplastics. *Ariz. Med.* **28**, 271–275.
2. Ignoffe, R.J. and Friedman, M.A. (1980). Therapy of local toxicities caused by extravasation of cancer chemotherapeutic drugs. *Can. Treat. Rev.* **7**, 17–27.
3. Maccara, M.E. (1983). Extravasation, a hazard of intravenous therapy. *Drug Intell. Clin. Pharm.* **17**, 713–717.
4. McNeece, J. and Lighty, J. (1986). *Cytotoxic extravasation manual*. Pharmacy Department, Leeds General Infirmary, Leeds.
5. Rudolph, R. and Larson, D.L. (1987). Etiology and treatment of chemotherapeutic agent extravasation injuries: a review. *J. Clin. Onc.* **5**, 1116–1126.

6. Slater, A. (1985). Extravasation of cytotoxic agents. *Can. Top.* 5, 52.
7. Anon. (1986). *Chemotherapy instruction manual*, 3rd Edn. Yorkshire Regional Cancer Organization, Cookridge Hospital, Leeds.
8. Pritchard, A.P. and David, J.A. Eds. (1988). *The Royal Marsden Hospital, Manual of clinical nursing procedures*, 2nd edn. Harper and Row, London.

CHAPTER 10

Home-based Cytotoxic Chemotherapy

INTRODUCTION

1 Potential Benefits of Home Chemotherapy

Chemotherapy is a major weapon in the treatment of a wide variety of cancers and may be used either as a single modality or in combination with radiotherapy and/or surgery. Traditionally, patients requiring chemotherapy have been admitted into hospital as in-patients or as day-case patients to receive their medication. Day-case treatment often requires the patient to be hospitalized for two or three days either because of protracted treatment regimens or because a combination of severe side-effects and the remote geographical location of the patient's home from the hospital preclude discharge until the patient is well enough to travel. This approach to cancer chemotherapy results in the patient spending considerable time away from home, from the work-place and from their family.

Understandably, it is the desire of most patients to be able to remain at home and to live as normal a life-style as possible.[1] Demand for home-based treatment combined with developments in drug administration technology have resulted in the emergence of domiciliary chemotherapy programmes where the patient is able to receive parenteral chemotherapy in his own home. Home-based chemotherapy not only reduces the stress and inconvenience of attending hospital but also enables the patient to take an active role in his treatment.

Home chemotherapy enables the patient to enjoy greater independence, particularly if the chemotherapy is self-administered. The active involvement of patients in their treatment tends to encourage a more positive attitude to chemotherapy. Drug-related side-effects may be more readily tolerated if patients are able to remain at home with their families in familiar surroundings.

Families of cancer patients often experience a feeling of helplessness and inadequacy but home-based treatment provides an opportunity for families and close friends to give assistance and support with treatment. All of these factors can contribute to increased morale of patients and their families. Psychological studies[2] on both domiciliary and hospitalized patients receiving similar chemotherapy regimens have demonstrated improved quality of life and a greater sense of well-being in the home-based group of patients. Home treatment also reduces the exposure of immunocompromised cancer patients to hospital infections.[1]

From an economical perspective, a properly managed, home chemotherapy programme can reduce costs associated with hospitalization and increase treatment availability. In a randomized study of in-patient versus out-patient continuous infusion chemotherapy for patients with locally advanced head and neck cancer, Vokes *et al*.[3] estimated a reduction in daily costs of $366 US per patient for domiciliary chemotherapy.

2 Potential Disadvantages and Limitations of Home Chemotherapy

In the home setting, professional assistance is not readily available to the patient. Acute drug-related toxicity, equipment failure, extravasation of the drug infusion and infection of the central venous catheter are difficulties which may cause patients severe distress. Acute toxicity can be minimized by using continuous ambulatory infusions for drug delivery and by pharmacodynamic individualization of drug dosage (*see* page 74). It is essential that patients are given thorough training on how to react in cases of equipment failure and that this is supported by written instructions and a 24-hour telephone number to enable home-based patients to contact a member of the oncology team. Most complications can be anticipated and dealing with them forms an integral part of the patient training programme. With experienced Home Care Oncology Teams, complications are rare and catheter infection rates of less than 1% are obtainable.[4]

It must also be accepted that some patients are not capable of maintaining their treatment at home. This may be because they are unable to understand basic instructions relating to their treatment or because of a physical disability (eg arthritis) that would prevent them from handling medication syringes and other equipment. In some cases support from family or friends may not be available and communications with the hospital-based Oncology team may be difficult (eg the patient may not have access to a telephone). Some patients may prefer the security of a hospital and are unwilling to take on the responsibility of home-based treatment. Careful patient selection is essential and will exert a profound influence on the outcome of home chemotherapy.

The economics of home chemotherapy may not always be viewed in a favourable light, largely because health care financial systems are inflexible and geared to in-patient treatment. Although home chemotherapy may release hospital beds, costs will actually increase if these are subsequently occupied by other patients. At best, home-based treatment provides hospital managers with a choice: either they can reduce the number of oncology beds and save money or they can re-occupy the released beds with other patients (not necessarily cancer patients) and reduce waiting lists. In addition, savings made at ward level may be difficult to transfer to the budgets of those departments (eg Pharmacy) where expenditure is increased as a result of home chemotherapy.

CLINICAL CONSIDERATIONS

1 Patient Selection

Careful patient selection is crucial to the success of a home chemotherapy programme. Before the option of domiciliary treatment is offered the clinician must establish that the patient is well motivated, physically capable of managing their medication syringes, infusion pump or other equipment and that the patient is able to understand detailed instructions. Normally, patients should have a reasonable performance status (Karnofsky score of at least 60) and should be capable of enjoying a satisfactory quality of life during home treatment. Ideally, support should be available from family and friends who are able to adjust or disrupt their own routines in order to help care for the patient. The availability of transport to and from the Oncology out-patient clinic must be considered and although it is possible to offer home chemotherapy to patients who live some distance from their hospital, access to a telephone is essential.

A wide range of cancers, including leukaemias (during remission) and solid tumours can be treated in the domiciliary setting. Patients with solid tumours of the breast, pancreas, colon, oesophagus and liver, often with metastatic disease, have been treated in the Home Oncology Programme, Exeter (HOPE) in the UK[4] and in similar programmes in the USA.[5,6] In many cases, home patients are being treated for recurrent disease following surgery or radiotherapy and the disease may be at an advanced stage. Patients in the late stages of disease or with fistulae, internal bleeding, ascites, systemic infection or severe nutritional deficiency are clearly not suitable for home treatment. Similarly, those patients who are unable to cope with the psychological and emotional stress associated with cancer should be offered the professional care available in the hospital or hospice system.

2 Dose Schedules

Bolus and short-term infusions

Although it is possible to administer home chemotherapy in traditional bolus or short-term infusion schedules, this approach is not always appropriate for domiciliary patients. In the hospital setting it is possible to control the acute toxicity (such as nausea and vomiting) associated with conventional chemotherapy. For domiciliary patients, such toxicity is more difficult to control and would be unacceptable. Conventional bolus or short-term infusion schedules would normally be administered by a community nurse. Some patients may feel that this restricts their freedom and independence, negating the advantages of home treatment over hospital day-case treatment.

In cases where experience has shown that bolus chemo-therapy is well tolerated, it may be possible to offer patients

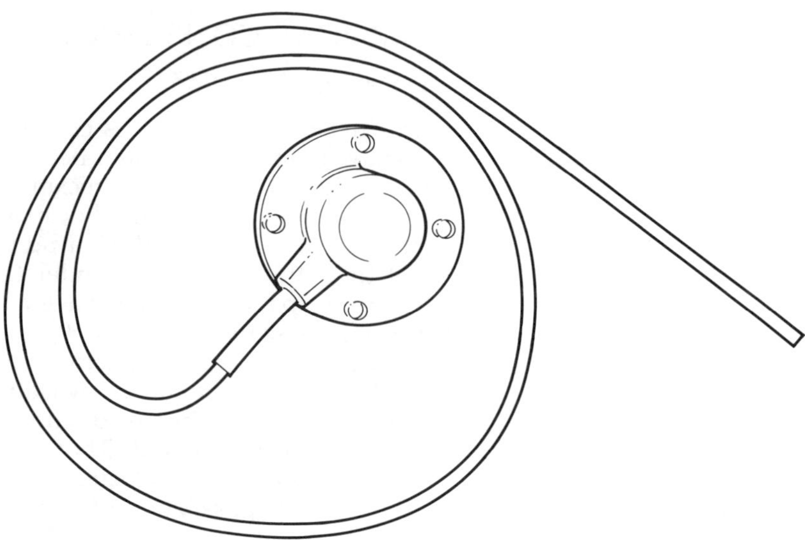

Figure 10.1: *Intraport Venous Access Port*

the option of self-medication by using a venous access device such as the Intraport shown in Figure 10.1. The catheter is inserted into a central vein (usually the subclavian vein) and the medication port is implanted subcutaneously, usually in the anterior chest wall, with the silastic septum located just beneath the skin. The septum is designed for multiple puncture and when not in use the patency of the system is maintained by flushing with dilute heparinized saline at monthly intervals.[7] Venous access devices provide a means of prolonged central venous access for cancer patients without frequent venipuncture and also for patients with difficult peripheral venous access as a result of obesity or emaciation. The safe administration of vesicant chemotherapy regimens is also made possible by these devices providing that the catheter is placed in a central vein.

The self-administration of small-volume subcutaneous injections may be appropriate for low-dose maintenance regimens providing that drug-related toxicity is minimal and the drug is non-vesicant. Home-care packs containing medication and the necessary syringes and needles are now available for this purpose (eg administration packs of interferon alfa-2a, Roche Products Ltd). Devices used to aid the subcutaneous administration of insulin to diabetic patients (eg the Novopen) may also be of benefit to leukaemia and cancer patients.

Prolonged continuous infusion

Attempts to improve the therapeutic index of antitumour drugs have focused on the replacement of traditional, rapid infusion schedules with prolonged continuous infusion regimens.[8] Recent developments with portable ambulatory infusion pumps have facilitated continuous infusion chemotherapy for domiciliary patients.

The rationale for continuous infusion chemotherapy is based on the pharmacokinetic characteristics of cytotoxic drugs and on the cytokinetic (growth cycle) profile of tumour cells.[8] Since many cytotoxic drugs have short plasma half-lives, continuous infusion regimens prolong the exposure of tumour cells to the drug. As tumour cells progress through the cell cycle, a greater proportion of the tumour cell population is exposed to the drug during the sensitive phase(s) of the cell cycle.

An additional advantage with continuous infusion regimens in home chemotherapy programmes is that adverse effects associated with peak plasma levels are reduced or eliminated. For example, doxorubicin is less cardiotoxic[9] and fluorouracil less myelosuppressive[10] in continuous infusion regimens. There is evidence that nausea and vomiting associated with bolus doses of cisplatinum are significantly reduced when infusional regimens are used.[11] However, other toxicities, such as mucositis and hand-foot syndrome in the case of fluorouracil,[12] may occur more readily with prolonged infusions.

Controlled studies[13,14] indicate that, on balance, drug-related adverse effects are reduced with infusional regimens and quality of life for the patient is improved. A study by Coates *et al.*[13] compared continuous infusion and intermittent bolus regimens in the home-based treatment of 308 patients with breast cancer. They reported only a marginal increase in efficacy with the continuous infusion regimen but there were statistically significant differences in toxicity and quality of life parameters, both in favour of continuous infusion. The authors concluded that continuous infusion was superior to the intermittent bolus schedule despite their declared hope to prove otherwise.[13]

LOGISTICAL CONSIDERATIONS

1 The Home Oncology Team

The success of home-based chemotherapy is dependent upon a team approach towards patient care. The Home Oncology Team would typically include a consultant Oncologist, Oncology Nurse and Oncology Pharmacist. If chemotherapy is to be administered as a continuous infusion using ambulatory pumps it will be necessary to include an experienced Anaesthetist in the team for the placement of central venous catheters. Similarly, if implantable venous access devices are to be used, the services of a Surgeon will be required. If home-based patients are receiving ambulatory continuous infusion chemotherapy at least one member of the team (usually the Pharmacist or Nurse) should be available 24 hours a day to deal with any problems that may arise with infusion pumps or the central venous catheter.

It is unlikely that the responsibility for home oncology treatment could be devolved to community-based health care professionals since cytotoxic chemotherapy should only be administered under the direction of an experienced Oncologist.

Also, the facilities and expertise required to prepare infusional cytotoxic medication reside within the hospital Pharmaceutical service, alongside other necessary support services including drug information and quality control.[4] The hospital-based team is also able to call upon the resources of other departments, such as Microbiology and Medical Electronics (for the testing and calibration of infusion pumps). If home chemotherapy is to be based on nurse-administered bolus or short infusion schedules, the team should contain a fully trained hospital-based, community Oncology Nurse. It is, of course, essential that the patient's general practitioner is informed of the treatment. If it becomes necessary to switch from chemotherapy to pain control, the venous access system used for chemotherapy can then be used for the infusion of opiates. In these cases, hospice Nurses may become involved in the preparation and administration of opiate infusions.

2 Venous Access Devices

Central venous catheters have been widely used for many years to deliver chemotherapy and total parenteral nutrition. These devices provide a reliable system for the administration of prolonged continuous infusions and, when attached to a venous access port, may also be used to deliver concentrated bolus injections of cytotoxic drugs to a central vein. The Hickman[15] and the smaller internal diameter, Broviac[16] catheters are suitable for ambulatory use and give rise to very few complications. Central venous catheters are normally placed in the subclavian vein and are tunnelled subcutaneously for a few centimetres at the site of entry to provide a barrier against the ingress of micro-organisms. A dacron cuff around the catheter just distal to the site of entry is used to hold the catheter in place. This cuff also helps to promote fibrosis of tissues at the site of catheter entry and this creates an additional barrier to micro-organisms. The site of catheter entry is further protected by an occlusive dressing which is changed at least fortnightly during visits to the Oncology out-patient's clinic. Between courses of chemotherapy, patency of the catheter is maintained by daily infusions of heparinized saline.

Care should be taken not to infuse drug combinations which may exhibit physical incompatibility and form precipitate in the central venous catheter. Double and triple lumen catheters are available for the infusion of multiple drug regimens. Although the central venous catheter could be used to aspirate blood samples this practice may increase the risk of venous thrombosis and is not to be recommended. Venous thrombosis may occur at any time when the catheter is in place. Thrombosis usually occurs near the catheter tip and is characterized by venous distension in the neck, swelling of the arm and pain in the shoulder, arm or neck.[17] The catheter itself may become occluded and resistance to flow may prevent the correct function of relatively low-powered ambulatory infusion pumps. Thrombosis secondary to the placement of a central venous catheter is a clear indication for immediate catheter removal. Infusions of thrombolytic agents such as urokinase have been used in an attempt to salvage the catheter but the efficacy and safety of this approach is controversial.[17]

Infection at the site of catheter entry is another potential complication, although with good clinical practice and expert catheter placement the incidence of this complication can be reduced to below 1%.[4] Infections at the site of catheter entry usually present as an abscess or cellulitis where the catheter enters the skin. Blood cultures from the site of entry and from a remote peripheral site should be carried out to characterize the infecting micro-organism and to exclude systemic infection. Superficial infections can be controlled with topical antibiotics and drainage, although systemic antibiotics may be required for neutropenic or febrile patients.[7] Infections involving the subcutaneous catheter tunnel usually necessitate removal of the catheter.

Instead of passing the central venous catheter out through the body for connection to an infusion pump, it may be connected to an implantable venous access port (Figure 10.1). These devices consist of a small-volume reservoir (usually 0.5 to 3 ml) and a silastic septum which is positioned subcutaneously. Venous access ports can be used to administer concentrated bolus injections which may prove vesicant to peripheral veins. Continuous infusions can also be administered via venous access ports by connecting the IV drug delivery tubing from the infusion pump to a 90° Huber needle. The Huber needle is then inserted through the skin into the septum of the venous access ports where it can be left in position for at least two weeks. When not in use the device is flushed with heparinized saline on a weekly basis.

Venous access ports are normally surgically implanted in the anterior chest wall. However, if the device is to be used for self-administration of bolus injections, it may be more convenient for the patient if the port is placed subcutaneously in the lower abdomen.

3 Ambulatory Infusion Pumps (*see* also Chapter 5)

A wide variety of ambulatory infusion pumps are now available, ranging in complexity from external syringe drivers to implantable, programmable pumps. For home chemotherapy, these devices must be safe, accurate and reliable and, in addition, should be lightweight, small and of rugged construction. Many of the external pump devices on the market meet these criteria and in most cases, external devices are perfectly adequate for ambulatory chemotherapy. Examples of two external infusion pumps, the Graseby, MS26 syringe driver and the programmable Parker, Micropump are shown in Figures 10.2 and 10.3 respectively. Both devices can be worn in a holster under the patient's clothing and both are relatively simple to operate. For details of the Graseby device, refer to Chapter 5.

For more specialized applications, programmable ambulatory pumps such as the Parker, Micropump (Figure 10.3) are now

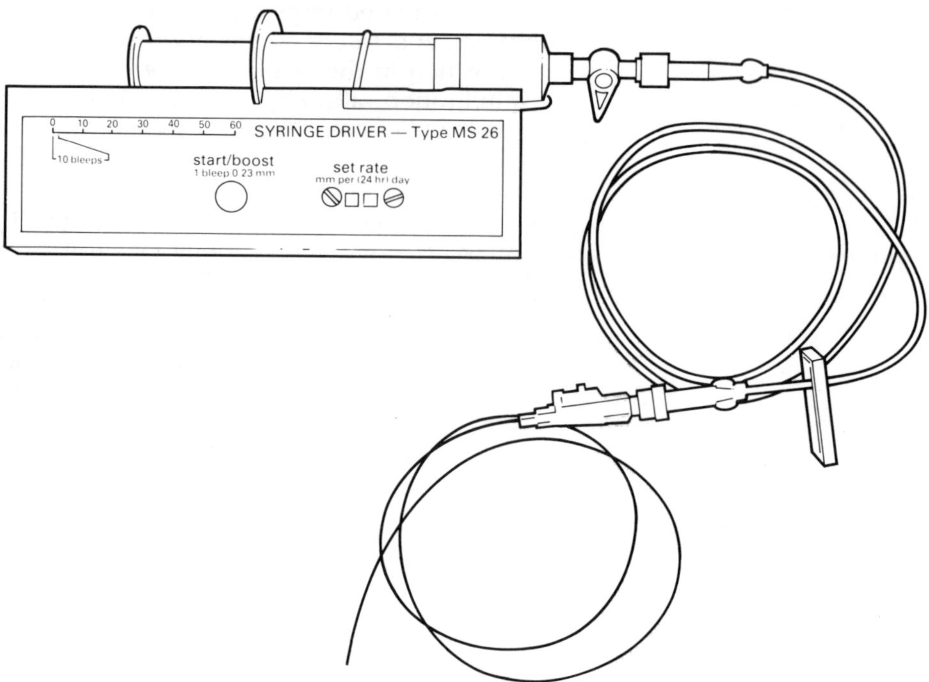

Figure 10.2: *Graseby, MS26 syringe driver together with central-venous catheter*

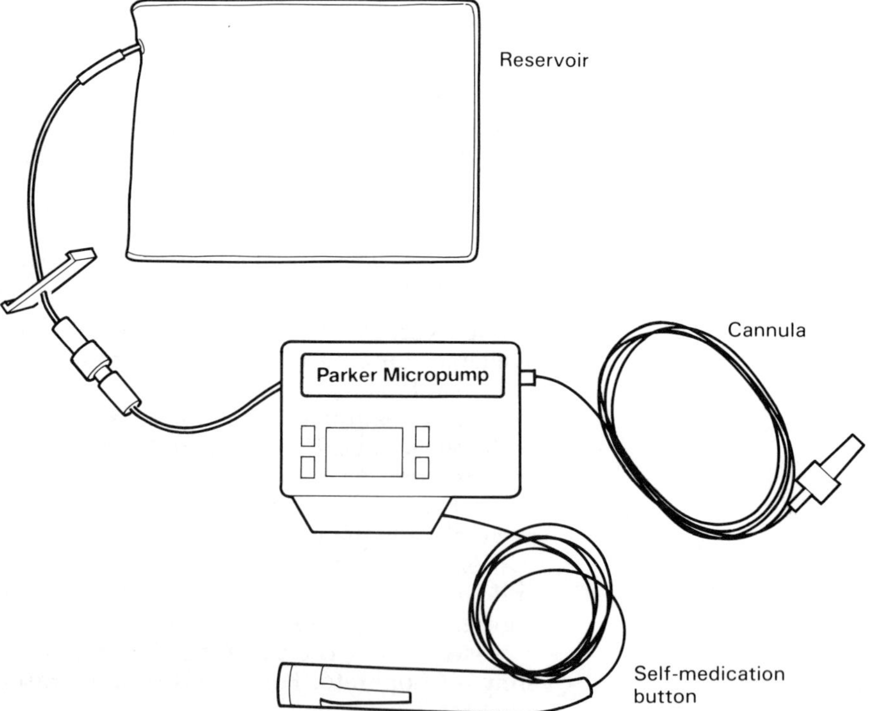

Figure 10.3: *Parker Micropump with infusion reservoir and 'pen-type' self-medication button*

available. The Parker Micropump weighs only 73 g and measures just 7.5 × 5 × 1.5 cm. The pump is worn in a waistband holster together with the medication reservoir which is a flat PVC pouch of either 100 ml or 200 ml capacity. The electromagnetically driven pumping mechanism is housed in a sealed cassette which is located in-line between the medication reservoir and the drug delivery catheter. The cassette can be removed from the pump and, because it forms part of a closed system with the catheter and medication reservoir, this feature enables the patient to bath, shower or even swim without damaging the pump mechanism.

The Parker Micropump contains its own microchip and is programmed from an external programming module. The programme is down-loaded into the internal memory of the pump which is then disconnected from the programming module. The Parker Micropump may be programmed to provide two different infusion rates and, therefore, lends itself to chronobiological studies where potential therapeutic advantages with circadian rhythm-based schedules have been reported.[18,19] The Parker Micropump also has a facility to allow the patient to self-inject medication boluses at a dosage and frequency defined by the programmer. This facility enables the pump to be used for ambulatory delivery of bolus chemotherapy and may also be used for pain control with infusions of opiates. The large medication reservoir of the Parker Micropump enables home treatment with poorly soluble drugs which, of necessity, are prepared in large volume infusions. The Micropump is powered by two silver oxide batteries which operate the pump mechanism and one lithium battery which maintains the memory back-up. Depending on the rate of infusion, the battery life is normally one to two weeks for the silver oxide batteries and up to six months for the lithium battery.

Examples of programmable, implantable, infusion pumps include the Infusaid (Shiley Infusaid Inc., USA) and the Synchromed (Medtronic Inc., USA) devices. The Synchromed pump is programmed externally through a radio-telemetry link.

For most home chemotherapy patients, simple syringe drivers are the infusion pump of choice. These are relatively cheap, reliable and easy to use. Syringe drivers use standard syringes with luer-lock fittings as the medication reservoir and, therefore, consumable costs are low. It is helpful to establish an ambulatory infusion pump policy within a hospital and to encourage the Home Oncology Team to use only one or two types of pump for home infusion. Staff with responsibility for training home patients in the use of infusion pumps will find their task much simpler if the range of pumps is limited. Also the range of consumables stocked and the range of spare parts held by the Medical Electronics Department will be more manageable.

4 Patient Procedures

Although specific to the HOPE programme, Exeter, UK[4,20] the patient procedures described in this section represent a typical approach followed by other home oncology centres.

Suitable patients are introduced to the concept of home chemotherapy (and prolonged continuous infusion, if appropriate) by the consultant Oncologist. If a patient decides to accept the option of home-based treatment he will then be referred to the Oncology Pharmacist for a more detailed explanation of the treatment. The patient is invited to view a video presentation, together with the Oncology Pharmacist, in which the consultant Oncologist and Oncology Pharmacist discuss various aspects of home chemotherapy with previously treated patients and their relatives. The video is produced by the Home Oncology Team and deals with specific issues of interest to the patient including insertion of the central venous catheter, changing of medication reservoirs, management of the infusion pump or venous access port and care of the dressing at the site of catheter entry. In the video presentation, previously treated patients discuss their treatment, their life-style and any difficulties they have encountered with the infusion pump. This often prompts the new patient to raise questions about the treatment and provides an opportunity for any anxieties or fears to be raised. The Oncology Pharmacist is required to take on the role of counsellor, a role that will be developed with each new patient as they attend the Oncology out-patients clinic at fortnightly intervals.

The patient is then admitted to the Oncology ward for a few days for insertion of the central venous catheter. This is an aseptic procedure and is carried out under local anaesthetic by an experienced Anaesthetist. Prior to discharge from hospital, the patient is trained in the management of their treatment by the Oncology Pharmacist. The patient is taught how to operate the infusion pump, how to recognize and respond to any warning alarms the pump may have, how to store medication reservoirs and change these in the pump when necessary. Instruction is given in the safe disposal of cytotoxic waste and used medication reservoirs. Often potential problems can be anticipated and are dealt with before they arise. For example, patients are often concerned by the presence of a small bubble of air in the infusion catheter. This is not clinically significant and the patient can be reassured before they even experience the problem themselves. Another problem that can occasionally occur is that the patient forgets to close the tap on the catheter before disconnecting the medication reservoir, resulting in venous blood flowing out through the catheter. Difficulties of this nature and the necessary action to take are always discussed with patients before they leave the hospital. The patient remains on the ward until the Pharmacist is satisfied that the patient is fully competent. This usually takes 24 to 48 hours. In some cases it may be advisable to train patients' relatives in the relevant techniques so that they are able to offer constructive support to the patient. As a back-up to the training programme, patients also receive concise written instructions and are given telephone numbers which may be used to contact Oncology Nurses or the Oncology Pharmacist, 24 hours a day.

On discharge from the hospital, the patient is supplied with pre-filled syringes or a medication reservoir for ambulatory pump use, or with pre-filled syringes for bolus injection. Where drug stability permits, the patient is supplied with sufficient medication for 14 days treatment (or if the treatment schedule is based on a period of less than 14 days, sufficient medication to complete the course). During breaks in chemotherapy, to permit bone marrow recovery, heparinized saline is supplied to ensure that the subclavian catheter remains patent. Examples of continuous infusion regimens used in the HOPE programme[4] are shown in Table 10.1 (*see* page 95).

The patient is also given supplies of consumables to take home with him. These include spare batteries for infusion pumps, protective gloves, sterile wipes for absorbing any minor spillage and burn-bins for disposing of cytotoxic waste and used syringes/medication reservoirs. A typical supply of consumables for a home chemotherapy patient is shown in Figure 10.4.

Patients attend the Oncology out-patient clinic once every two weeks where they are seen by the consultant Oncologist who monitors the patient's clinical condition. The dressing at the site of catheter entry is changed by the Oncology Nurse and the

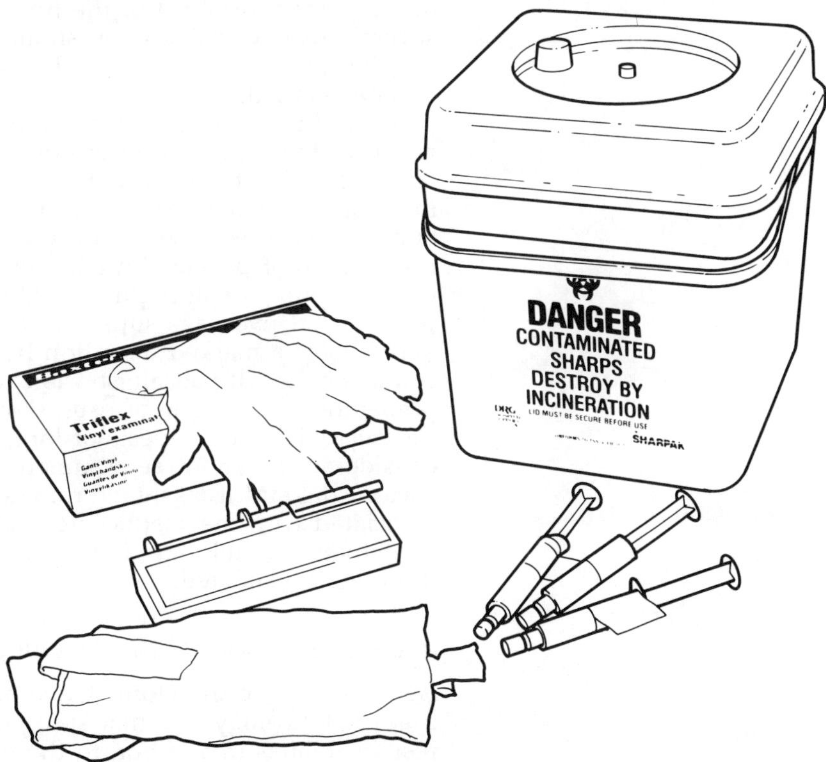

Figure 10.4: *Consumables supplied to home chemotherapy patients: burn-bin, gloves, infusion pump, spare battery, pump holster and pre-filled syringes*

Oncology Pharmacist is on hand to deal with any infusion pump-related problems or queries concerning adverse effects from the medication. During these fortnightly visits, patients collect further supplies of consumables from the out-patient clinic and further supplies of medication from the hospital Pharmacy.

Many patients participating in home chemotherapy programmes will be entered into controlled clinical trials, usually of a phase II or phase III nature. Visits to the out-patient clinic provide the Clinician with an opportunity to monitor the patient extensively and to determine the quality of life enjoyed by the patient during treatment. If pharmacokinetic studies also form part of the trial, it is preferable for blood samples to be taken by a visiting Oncology Nurse (or Pharmacist trained in phlebotomy), rather than subject the patient to repeated hospital visits.

PHARMACEUTICAL CONSIDERATIONS

1 Preparation of Medication for Home Chemotherapy Patients

The introduction of a home chemotherapy programme is likely to affect the work-load of the hospital Pharmacy department in several areas. Consideration should be given to resource and funding implications before a home chemotherapy programme is implemented.

Unless the number of hospital-based Oncology beds is reduced, the introduction of home chemotherapy may result in an increased patient throughput. This would be reflected by increased demands for the preparation of cytotoxic infusions and increased expenditure on the drugs budget. The preparation of pre-filled medication reservoirs for ambulatory infusion pumps will require additional staff training. The provision of five days supply of medication to home patients necessitates a marked deviation from the ideal practice of commencing drug administration within 24 hours of preparation. The issue of drug stability is addressed below but the microbiological aspects of long-term supply must also be considered. It cannot be assumed that cytotoxic infusions are bactericidal and it is, therefore, essential that all equipment associated with the aseptic preparation of medication for home patients is carefully monitored, and that all procedures are thoroughly validated.

2 Extended Role of the Oncology Pharmacist

As a member of the Home Chemotherapy Team it is essential that the Oncology Pharmacist is prepared to accept new responsibilities in addition to the traditional functions of drug preparation and distribution. The hospital Pharmacy department is an excellent centre for the co-ordination of the home chemotherapy programme.[1] The Oncology Pharmacist requires a detailed knowledge of infusion pumps, catheters and venous access ports to enable him to make sound recommendations on the type of ambulatory infusion system for each individual patient. The Pharmacist should have a clear understanding of stability and compatibility issues so that Clinicians can be made aware of both the possibilities and limitations of home chemotherapy regimens. As an educator, the Pharmacist's role would include the preparation of training material, training patients, training other health care professionals and liaising with health care workers outside the hospital setting.

3 Drug Stability and Compatibility

For most cytotoxic drugs, some recommendations on drug stability and compatibility are available from the manufacturers and are published in the *Data sheet compendium*.[21] However, these recommendations are restricted to licensed regimens which are invariably bolus injections or short-term infusions. In the case of home chemotherapy it must be recognized that even pre-filled syringes for bolus medication may be stored in the patient's refrigerator for several weeks before use. Drug infusions delivered by ambulatory pumps are not only stored for long periods (up to 14 days) under refrigerated conditions before use but are also subjected to temperatures of 35–37°C in the pump reservoir which is worn under the patient's clothing. It is, therefore, essential to determine the physical and chemical stability of infusions used in home chemotherapy regimens under both storage (4–8°C) and 'in-use' (35–37°C) conditions. Exposure times will vary according to the type of infusion pump used. Pre-filled syringes used in the Graseby syringe driver contain 24 hours supply of medication and are changed daily by the patient. If it is proposed to give 14 days supply of medication at a time, stability studies should be carried out under storage conditions (4–8°C) over 14 days and under in-use conditions (35–37°C) over 24 hours. In the case of infusion pumps with large volume cassettes or pouch-type medication reservoirs which contain sufficient infusion for five to 14 days treatment (depending on the regimen), drug stability under in-use conditions (35–37°C) should be determined over the treatment period. Since medication cassettes/pouches are normally connected to the infusion pump within 24 hours of preparation, stability studies under storage conditions (4–8°C) need only be continued over 24 hours. If, however, two pre-filled medication cassettes/pouches are supplied to give a total of 14 days treatment, drug stability would be determined over seven days under both storage and in-use conditions. It is advisable to monitor the temperature of each patient's own refrigerator to ensure that medication is stored at the correct temperature.

In view of the limited information available on the pharmacology and toxicology of degradation products arising from cytotoxic drugs, only fully validated stability-indicating assay methods should be used in chemical stability studies.

All stability investigations should be carried out on infusions in the type of syringe or medication reservoir to be used clinically. Weight changes of infusions should be monitored during storage, particularly at 37°C, since moisture loss from medication reservoirs can mask a reduction in drug assay arising from degradation.[22] Chemical stability data for some cytotoxic drug infusions in a variety of pump reservoirs are presented in Table 2.[23,24] Only interferon alpha-2a, which degrades by the cleavage of intra-molecular bonds and subsequent dimer formation was found to be unstable in infusion regimens.[25] Before a new type of medication reservoir or catheter is used for the first time, the level of extractives released from the plastic into the infusion should be determined. Plasticizer levels (as diethylhexylphthalate) extracted into infusions from medication reservoirs are low with typical concentrations of less than 1 µg/ml.[23] Care should be taken when using concentrated infusions of cytotoxic drugs formulated in co-solvent solutions (eg etoposide) since these can react with certain plastics causing hair-line cracks.[26]

THE PHARMACIST'S ROLE IN FUTURE DEVELOPMENTS

Most hospital Pharmacists who have worked with a Home Oncology Team have found the experience both rewarding and challenging. Both practice and research aspects of home-based oncology have required Pharmacists to develop and use their scientific, clinical and counselling skills at the highest level. Future developments in Home Oncology treatment will also require a significant Pharmaceutical input. Recent chronobiological studies[17,18] have suggested that administration of chemotherapy in accordance with circadian rhythms may reduce drug-related toxicity and improve the outcome of treatment. Dose calculations based on pharmacodynamic parameters[27] may also help in the control of adverse effects. Both approaches offer considerable potential for home chemotherapy treatment, where avoidance of severe drug toxicity is essential. These new developments require the modification and control of drug delivery systems and will clearly be dependent upon the availability of Pharmaceutical expertise.

Table 10.1: *Examples of ambulatory continuous infusion regimens used in the HOPE programme*[4]

Infusion	Dose Rate	Duration of each Course
Carboplatin	25 mg/day	5 days with synchronous radiotherapy
Doxorubicin	5 mg/day	30 days
5-Fluorouracil	500 mg/day	Continuous until side effects
Ifosfamide + Mesna	1 g + 1 g/day	10 days
Mitozantrone	2 mg/day	14 days

Table 10.2: *Chemical stability data for continuous infusion regimens under storage and in-use conditions* [23,25]

Infusion	Reservoir	Storage Time Temp. (°C)	Drug Assay (% of initial)	
Carboplatin (10 mg/ml)	Syringe (a)	5 days/4–8°	100.7	
		24 hours/37°	96.9	
	Medication pouch (b)	7 days/4–8°	101.0	
		7 days/37°	102.0	
Cytarabine (34 mg/ml)	Syringe (a)	14 days/4–8°	98.5	
		24 hours/37°	98.2	
Fluorouracil (25 mg/ml)	Syringe (a)	14 days/4–8°	100.1	
		24 hours/37°	98.3	
	Medication pouch (b)	7 days/4–8°	97.9	
		7 days/37°	99.1	
Epirubicin (8 mg/ml)	Medication cassette (c)	24 hours/4–8°	99.3	
		5 days/37°	102.9	
			(Ifos)	*(Mesna)*
Ifosfamide/ Mesna (50 mg/ml of each)	Syringe (a)	14 days/4–8°	99.4	99.4
		24 hours/37°	98.2	97.1
Interferon Alpha-2a (3 Mu/6 ml)	Syringe (a)	14 days/4–8°	unstable	
		24 hours/37°	unstable	
Mitozantrone (2 mg/ml)	Medication pouch (b)	7 days/4–8°	98.5	
		7 days/37°	95.7	

a) Polypropylene syringes 'Plastipak', Becton Dickinson.
b) Medication pouch for Parker Micropump, Parker Abbot.
c) Medication Cassette for Pharmacia, Deltec (CADD-1 pump), Pharmacia Inc.

See individual drug monographs for more detail.

REFERENCES

1. Bacovsky, R.A. (1988). *Home parenteral chemotherapy programs.* Proceedings of 1st international symposium on oncology pharmacy practice. New Zealand Hospital Pharmacists' Association, 294–300.
2. Payne, S. (1989). *Quality of life in women with advanced breast cancer.* PhD Thesis, Department of Psychology, University of Exeter.
3. Vokes, E.E. *et al.* (1989). A randomized study of in-patient versus out-patient continuous infusion chemotherapy for patients with locally advanced head and neck cancer. *Cancer,* **63**, 30–36.
4. Sewell, G.J. *et al* (1989). Home-based cancer therapy by continuous infusion. *Pharm. J.* **243**, 139–141.
5. Ausman, R.K. *et al.* (1982). Long-term, ambulatory, continuous intravenous Infusion of 5-fluorouracil for the treatment of metastatic adenocarcinoma in the liver. *Wisc. Med. J.* **81**, 25–28.
6. Lokich, J.J. *et al.* (1982). The delivery of cancer chemotherapy by constant venous infusion: ambulatory management of venous access and portable pump. *Cancer,* **50** (12), 2731–2735.
7. Finley, R.S. (1988). Ambulatory infusion pumps and venous access devices. Proceedings of 1st international symposium on oncology pharmacy practice. New Zealand Hospital Pharmacists' Association, 279–293.
8. Lokich, J.J. (1987). Introduction to the concept and practice of infusion chemotherapy. In Lokich, J.J. (ed.). *Can. Chemo. by Inf.* Precept Press Inc., Chicago, 3–11.
9. Legha, S.S. *et al.* (1982). Reduction of doxorubicin cardiotoxicity by prolonged continuous intravenous infusion. *Ann. Int. Med.* **96**, 133–139.
10. Seifert, P. *et al.* (1975). Comparison of continuously infused 5-fluorouracil with bolus injection in treatment of patients with colorectal adenocarcinoma. *Cancer,* **36**, 123–128.
11. Thigpen, J.T. (1989). A randomized comparison of a rapid versus prolonged (24 hr) infusion of cisplatin therapy of squamous cell carcinoma of the uterine cervix: a gynecologic oncology study. *Gyn. Onc.* **32**, 198–202.
12. Mortimer, J. and Anderson, I. (1989). Managing the toxicities unique to high-dose leukovorin (CF) and fluorouracil (FU). *Proc. Amer. Soc. Clin. Onc.* **8**, 98.
13. Coates, A. *et al.* (1987). Improving the quality of life during chemotherapy for advanced breast cancer. A comparison of intermittent and continuous treatment strategies. *New Eng. J. Med.* **317** (24), 1490–1495.
14. Lokich, J.J. *et al.* (1989). Prospective randomized comparison of continuous infusion fluorouracil with a conventional bolus schedule in metastatic colorectal carcinoma; a mid-Atlantic oncology program study. *J. Clin. Onc.* **7**, 425–432.

15. Hickman, R.O. *et al.* (1979) A modified right atrial catheter for access to the venous system in marrow transplant recipients. *Surg. Gynecol. Obstet.* **148**, 871–875.
16. Broviac, J.W. *et al.* (1973). A silicone rubber atrial catheter for prolonged parenteral alimentation. *Surg. Gynecol. Obstet.* **136**, 602–606.
17. Moor, C.L. (1987). Nursing management of infusion catheters. In: Lokich, J.J. (Ed.). *Cancer chemotherapy by infusion*, Precept Press Inc., Chicago. 64–74.
18. Hrushesky, W.J.M. (1983). The clinical application of chronobiology to oncology. *Am. J. Ant.* **168**, 519–542.
19. Von Roemeling, R., and Hrushesky, W.J.M. (1989). Circadian patterning of continuous floxuridine infusion reduces toxicity and allows higher dose intensity in patients with widespread cancer. *J. Clin. Onc.* **7**, 1710–1719.
20. Sewell, G.J. *et al.* (1987). HOPE for cancer. *J. Dist. Nur.* April, 4–6.
21. Anon. (1989). *ABPI Data Sheet Compendium, 1989–90.* Datapharm Publications Ltd, London.
22. Sewell, G.J. *et al.*(1987). The Stability of carboplatin in ambulatory continuous infusion regimes. *J. Clin. Pharm,* **12**, 427–432.
23. Sewell, G.J. (1988). Cancer chemotherapy by infusion, drug stability and compatibility considerations. Proceedings of 1st international symposium on oncology pharmacy practice. New Zealand Hospital Pharmacists' Association, 253–278.
24. Sewell, G.J. *et al.* (1988). Pharmaceutical aspects of domiciliary continuous infusion chemotherapy. *Brit. J. Cancer,* **58**, 536.
25. Palmer, A.J. (1988). Qualitative studies on α-interferon-2b in prolonged continuous infusion regimes using gradient elution high performance liquid chromatography. *J. Clin. Pharm. Ther.* **13**, 225–231.
26. Schwinghammer, T.L. and Reilly, M. (1988). Cracking of ABS plastic devices used to infuse undiluted etoposide injection (letter). *Am. J. Hosp. Pharm.* **45** (6), 1277.
27. Belani, C.P. *et al.* (1989). A novel pharmacodynamically-based approach to dose optimization of carboplatin when used in combination with etoposide. *J. Clin. Onc.* **7**, 1896–1902.

Storage of Cytotoxic Drugs After Reconstitution or Repackaging

Many parenteral cytotoxics require reconstitution. In a centralized service, cytotoxic injections will normally be drawn up into a syringe or into an infusion container ready for administration. Manufacturers are currently required by licensing authorities to indicate on the Data Sheet and package insert that reconstituted drugs, with or without preservative, should be stored in a refrigerator (unless dictated by the chemical nature of the drug) and must be used within a specified period, usually not more than 24 hours. This is to ensure that, although the drug may be stable, any micro-organisms introduced during the reconstitution procedures (assumed to be on the ward) will have insufficient opportunity to multiply and reach hazardous numbers before the injection is administered.

This recommendation or directive, therefore, will not usually relate to considerations of chemical stability. Consequently, provided that any manipulations undertaken to prepare the drug for administration are carried out under aseptic conditions, ensuring that an adequate level of sterility assurance is maintained, the shelf-life of such reconsitituted or repackaged injections can be extended at the discretion of the responsible hospital Pharmacist.

It is essential that good aseptic techniques are employed and adequate Quality Assurance programmes maintained. The shelf-life of such injectables can then be governed by chemical stability considerations together with local practice and procedures. This allows far greater flexibility and opportunities for greater efficiency in operating centralized cytotoxic services.

Guidance in each Monograph regarding storage after reconstitution assumes that subsequent manipulations are undertaken under appropriate aseptic conditions. The Monographs have been prepared from reviews of the literature, guidance from the respective manufacturer and the author's own studies and experience. However, responsibility for the final preparation must rest with the Pharmacist responsible for the cytotoxic services.

These Monographs describe injectable cytotoxics used widely in the UK, USA, Australasia and Europe. Information has, wherever possible, been referenced to specific sources of information. Data and information from the particular manufacturer may originate from a variety of sources, including Data Sheets, package inserts and personal communications, held on file by the author of the Monograph. A glossary of drug names and product titles used in different countries is included for reference purposes.

Each Monograph has a common structure for ease of reference and uniformity. The purpose of each section is described below. The major aim in producing the Monographs is to provide the user with all the available information for each injection concerning stability in the context of a cytotoxic service operated by a Pharmacy department.

1 General Details

Under the heading Approved names, the first name(s) refers to INNM titles, followed by alternatives in common use.

As well as nomenclature, this section includes manufacturers and suppliers in the UK. Details for other countries are included in the Glossary (pp. 163).

2 Chemistry

A summary of the chemical properties of the drug relevant to the injection form (structure, solubility, etc.).

3 Stability Profile

A summary of the chemical stability of each drug is given, including chemical and physical parameters that influence stability after reconstitution and repackaging. Degradation pathways, when known, are included as background information. Important practical aspects, including container compatibility, known incompatibilities with other drugs and a summary of the stability of the reconstituted injection, complete this section.

4 Clinical Use

A brief summary of dosage regimens commonly used are included for guidance purposes only.

5 Preparation of Injection

Details of how the injection is prepared for bolus injection and infusion, as relevant, are included, together with handling precautions and details concerning treatment of extravasation. Information concerning specific references to gloves recommended for handling originates from the manufacturer or the literature. It is generally considered, however, that the material used to make the glove is less important than glove thickness. For further guidance, see Chapter 3.

6 Destruction of Drug or Contaminated Articles

The recommended methods of inactivating each cytotoxic drug are summarized under the headings Incineration, Chemical, and Contact with skin. The incineration conditions indicate the minimum temperatures recommended, usually by the manufacturer. *See* Chapter 6 for more details concerning safe handling.

> NOTE: While the authors of each Monograph have taken every care to provide accurate and complete information, as far as it is possible to do so, the authors or publishers cannot accept any liability for the information therein.

AMSACRINE

1 General Details

Approved names: Amsacrine, AMSA, m-AMSA.

Proprietary name: Amsidine Concentrate for Infusion.

Manufacturer or supplier: Parke-Davis Research Laboratories Ltd.

Presentation and formulation details: Orange/red solution of amsacrine in 2 ml ampoules containing 1.5 ml injection, 50 mg/ml amsacrine. The diluent vial contains 13.5 ml of 0.0353 M/L lactic acid solution. Amsacrine is dissolved in anhydrous N.N-dimethylacetamide (DMA). The diluent vial contains lactic acid in order to form the lactate salt of amsacrine when the drug is added to the diluent, under the acid conditions prevailing. The presence of DMA also prevents the formation of gelatinous material normally seen in aqueous amsacrine lactate solutions.

Storage and shelf-life of unopened container: Three years at ambient temperature not exceeding 25°C.

2 Chemistry

Type: Acridine-like DNA intercalating agent.

Molecular structure:
4'-(Acridine-9-ylamino)methanesulphon-*m*-anisidine.

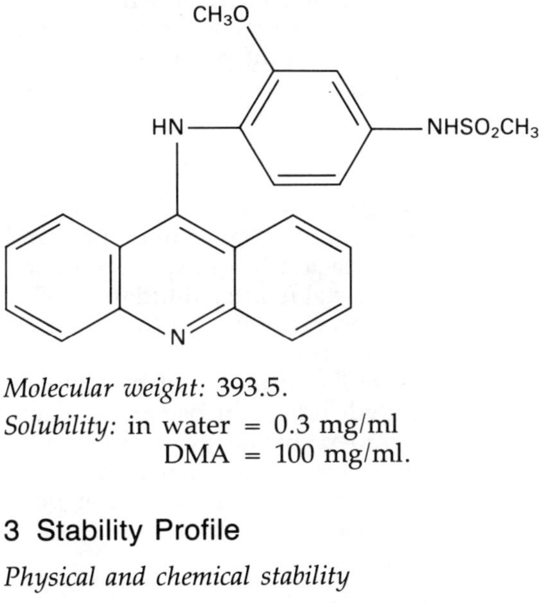

CH₃O

HN— —NHSO₂CH₃

N

Molecular weight: 393.5.

Solubility: in water = 0.3 mg/ml
DMA = 100 mg/ml.

3 Stability Profile

Physical and chemical stability

Amsacrine is relatively stable in an aqueous vehicle, provided reconstitution takes place in the presence of lactate ions, and pH remains acid. It is stable for 48 hours after dilution in 5% dextrose.[1] As the drug is incompatible with chloride or sulphate ions, saline must be avoided as a diluent. The hydrochloride salt of amsacrine is poorly water soluble.

Degradation pathways: 9(10H)-acridone, 9-chloroacridine and 4-aminomethanesulphon-m-amsidine are formed as degradation products.

Physical stability is not significantly affected by normal temperature ranges. The drug is light-sensitive. After dilution in 5% dextrose at a final concentration of 150 µg/ml, amsacrine is stable during exposure to diffuse daylight or fluorescent light over a 48 hour period.[1] Since amsacrine solutions are relatively insoluble in water, DMA is included in the drug diluent to prevent precipitation when the drug is reconstituted.

It has been reported that DMA may increase extraction of components of rubber or certain plastic material.[2] Consequently, it is recommended that only glass syringes should be employed to transfer the drug concentrate to the diluent vial and from vial to infusion. However, this study examined only leaching from PVC infusion containers and administration sets. Most plastic syringes are composed of polypropylene barrels with rubber plungers so this study is not relevent. The company points out that studies using the amsacrine/DMA solution in polypropylene syringes were not conclusive in demonstrating elution of these substances; however, contamination with such chemicals may affect the stability and toxicity profile of amsacrine and glass syringes should be used for the initial steps in the preparation of the infusion. Once diluted in 500 ml 5% glucose, however, DMA is sufficiently dilute not to interact with plastic infusion containers, sets or lines.[3] One other problem that can arise is the effect of DMA on the physical performance characteristics of syringes. Experience indicates that amsacrine concentrate does not affect the physical performance of polypropylene syringes.

Compatibility information: No further information available.

Stability in clinical practice

The reconstituted drug is stable in the diluent provided for 48 hours at room temperature and ambient lighting. It should be protected from exposure to strong daylight. Amsacrine is also stable after dilution in 5% glucose for 48 hours (at concentrations up to 800 µg/ml, data supplied by the manufacturer).

Amsacrine must not be diluted in saline infusions.[4] Amsacrine diluted in 5% glucose at a concentration of 150 µg/ml is not degraded during exposure to diffuse daylight or fluorescent light over a 48-hour period.[3] It was also reported that amsacrine was not absorbed by PVC or polybutadiene-containing administration sets.[3]

4 Clinical Use

Type of cytotoxic: Inhibitor of DNA.

Main indications: Acute leukaemia.

Dosage: Induction – 90 mg/m² day for five days. Maintenance – 50 mg/m² day for 3 days.

5 Preparation of Injection

Dilution: Transfer 1.5 ml of amsacrine solution in DMA (in the ampoule) to the diluent vial, preferably using a glass syringe. The resulting solution contains 5 mg/ml amsacrine.

Bolus administration: Not recommended.

Infusion: Add required volume of diluted amsacrine to 500 ml 5% glucose infusion. Infuse over 60 to 90 minutes. Problems of phlebitis are more likely with higher concentrations and the data sheet recommends dilution of 75 mg amsacrine in 500 ml 5% glucose solution.[4]

Gloves for handling: Polyethylene.

Extravasation: Very damaging; no known antidote. Apply ice-pack to affected area.

6 Destruction of Drug or Contaminated Articles

Incineration: 260°C.

Chemical: 10% sodium hypochlorite/24 hours.

Contact with skin: wash with soap and water.

References

1. D'Arcy, P.F. (1983). Reactions and interactions in handling anticancer drugs. *Drug Intell. Clin. Pharm.* **17**, 532–538.
2. Vishnuvajjala, R.B. and Cradock, J.C. (1984). Compatibility of plastic infusion devices with diluted N-Methyl-Formamide and N.N.-dimethylacetamide. *Am. J. Hosp. Pharm.* **41**, 1160–1163.
3. Cartwright-Shamoon, J.M. *et al.* (1988). Examination of sorption and photodegradation of amsacrine in intravenous burette administration sets. *In. J. Pharm.* **42**, 41–46.
4. ABPI Data Sheet Compendium 1989–90. (1989). Datapharm Publications Ltd, London, pp. 1184–1185.

Prepared by M.C. Allwood

ASPARAGINASE

1 General Details

Approved names: Crisantaspase, Erwinia L-asparaginase.

Proprietary name: Erwinase.

Manufacturer or supplier: Porton Products Ltd.

Presentation and formulation details: White, freeze-dried powder in 2 ml rubber-capped vials containing 10 000 IU asparaginase. Each pack contains 20 vials.

Inactive ingredients: Glucose 5.0 mg, sodium chloride 0.6 mg. 1 IU Crisantaspase releases 1 μmol ammonia/minute from L-asparagine.

Storage and shelf-life of unopened container: Three years at 2 to 8°C.[1]

2 Chemistry

Type: Bacterial enzyme protein from Erwinia chrysanthemi.
Molecular weight: 130,000.
Activity: 700 U/mg.
Solubility in water: Highly soluble.[2]

3 Stability Profile

Physical and chemical stability

Stable in solution for at least 20 days at 37°C. Denaturation of the protein and loss of enzyme activity occur outside physiological pH range (6–7.5).[3]

Degradation pathways: No information available.

Physical: Polymerization of the reconstituted enzyme solution occurs after 15 minutes. Gelatinous fibres are produced. Enzyme activity is retained. Polymerization is initiated by contact with the rubber closure of the vial.[3]

Container compatibility: Stable in glass containers or syringes, avoid contact with rubber. No data on stability in plastic syringes, but most syringes contain a rubber plunger.

Compatibility with other drugs: Should not be mixed with other drugs.

Stability in clinical practice

Solutions should be administered as soon as possible after reconstitution since contact with the rubber stopper denatures the reconstituted drug and forms minute filaments of insoluble material. The effect, however, is not progressive and does not affect the potency of the solution. Sterile solutions transferred to glass syringes retain potency for at least 20 days at 37°C.[1]

4 Clinical Use

Type of cytotoxic: Therapeutic enzyme – not a true cytotoxic agent.

Main indications: Used in combination with other agents in treatment of acute lymphatic leukaemia and some other neoplastic conditions.

Dosage: 200 IU/kg body-weight (5,000–6,000 IU/m^2 body-surface area) by intramuscular injection three times per week for nine doses.[3] Also refer to current MRC protocols.

5 Preparation of Injection

Reconstitution: The contents of the vial should be reconstituted with 1 to 2 ml of 0.9% sodium chloride injection and dissolved with gentle mixing to avoid contact with the rubber stopper.

Administration: The intramuscular route is preferred as it is associated with the fewest toxic effects. The solution may also be given by subcutaneous injection. Intravenous injection or infusion is rarely indicated but may be used if necessary.

Infusion: Administration by infusion is not usually necessary. Asparaginase is stable for at least seven days in solution in 0.9% sodium chloride and 5% glucose.[2] Enzyme activity may be adversely affected if the pH of the solution is outside the normal physiological range.[3]

Gloves for handling: Rubber gloves should be worn. Although not a cytotoxic, the agent may cause sensitivity reactions.

Extravasation: Administration is usually by intramuscular or subcutaneous injection. No harmful local effects will result from extravasation of solutions given intravenously.

6 Destruction of Drug or Contaminated Articles

Incineration: 800°C.

Chemical: Strong acids or alkalis will denature the protein.

Contact with skin: Wash with water.

References

1. ABPI Datasheet Compendium 1989/90. (1989). Datapharm Publications Ltd, London, p. 1273.
2. Wade, H.E. (1986). *Development of Erwinase (Erwinia Asparaginase).* Lecture to symposium: Erwinia Asparaginase in the treatment of leukaemia. Frankfurt, Germany. 21 November 1986.
3. Porton Products Ltd, (1988). Data on file. Porton Products Limited, Centre for Applied Microbiological Research. Porton Down, Salisbury, Wiltshire SP4 0JG.

Prepared by J.M. Oakes

AZACYTIDINE

1 General Details

Approved name: Azacytidine, Ladakamycin.

Proprietary name: Mylosar.

Manufacturer or supplier: Upjohn Limited, Pharmaceutical Division.

Presentation and formulation details: Lyophilized powder, 100 mg azacytidine with 100 mg mannitol in a 20 ml vial.

Storage and shelf-life of unopened container: Four years at 2 to 8°; two years at 25°C.

2 Chemistry

Type: Inhibitor of DNA.

Molecular structure: 4-amino-1-D-ribofuranosyl-1,2,4 triazin-2(1H)-one.

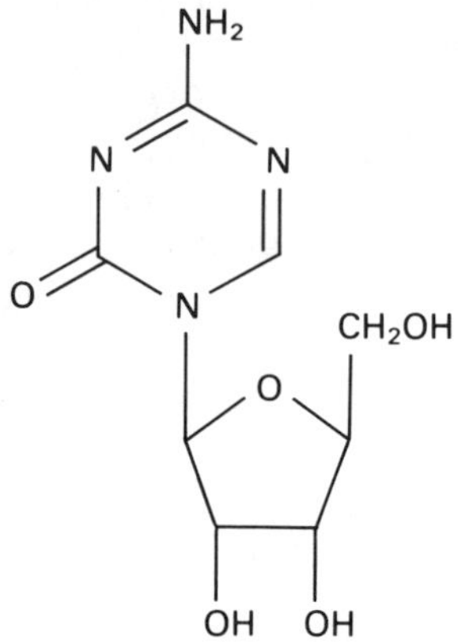

Molecular weight: 244.2.

3 Stability Profile

Physical and chemical stability

Azacytidine is rapidly hydrolyzed in water. In neutral and alkaline solutions it undergoes hydrolytic cleavage across the 5–6 bond to give β-D ribofuranosyl-3-guanylurea (II) via the labile intermediate N-formyl-ribosylguanylurea (I). In strong acid the glycosidic linkage is cleaved to give D-ribose, 5-azacytidine (III) and 5-azauracil (IV), the latter two undergoing further hydrolysis and ring cleavage to give various non-chromophoric products (*see* Figure 1).

The kinetics of the hydrolysis reactions are complex making stability prediction difficult.[1] Neutral solutions of azacytidine are most stable, with the maximum stability being in the pH range of 6.5–7.0.[1,2] Consequently, in infusion fluids the drug is least stable in glucose solutions and most stable in lactated Ringer's solution.[3] In unbuffered solutions, the pH of 2 mg/ml solutions is about 6.5 whereas the pH of 0.2 mg/ml solution is very much lower (4.5–5.5). Solutions of the drug are, therefore, more stable at the higher concentration. The $T_{90\%}$ does not exceed three hours in any solution. In 5% glucose the $T_{90\%}$ for 0.2 mg/ml solutions is as low as 45 minutes.

Stability in clinical practice

Solutions containing 2 mg/5 ml may be stored for three hours but caution is required below this concentration. Dilutions in 5% glucose must be administered within one hour of preparation,

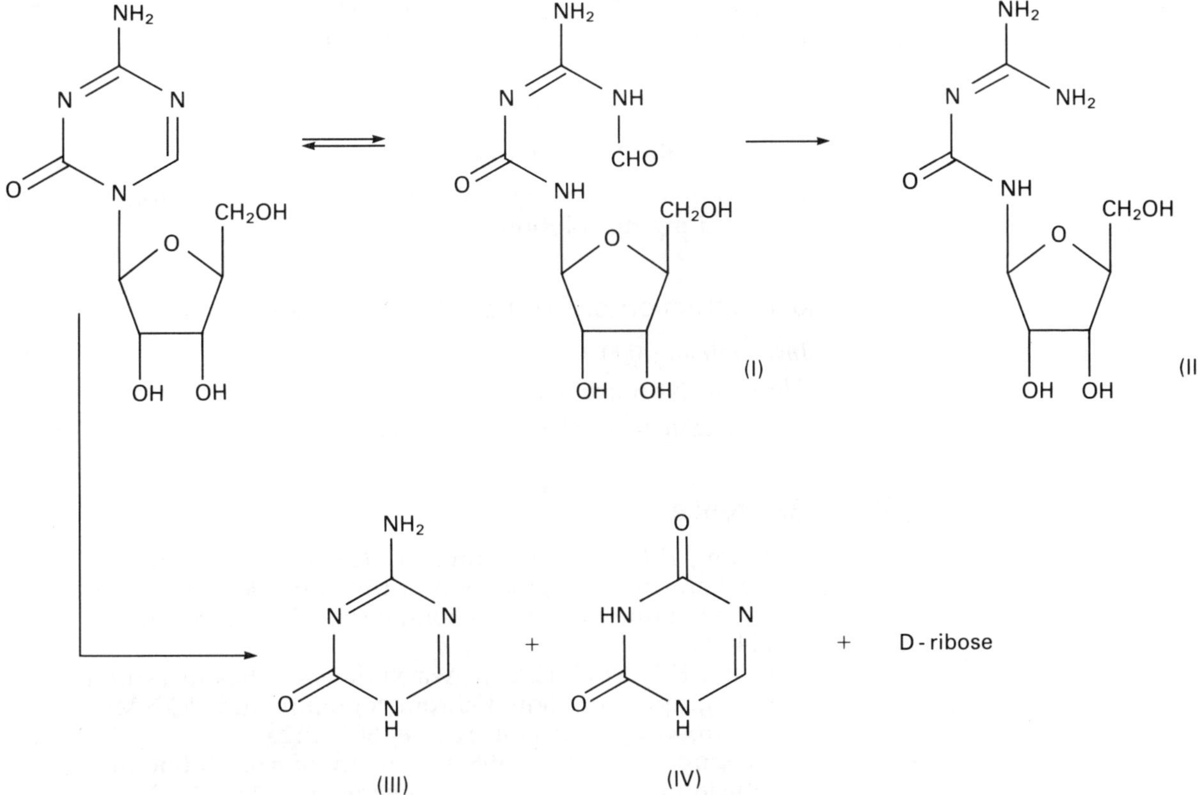

Figure 1: *Degradation pathways for azacytidine*

unless buffered to pH 6.5–7.0. In the presence of a five to ten-fold excess of sodium bisulphite, at pH 2.5, azacytidine forms an addition product with the bisulphite and is consequently stable for up to 20 hours at ambient temperatures, or four days at 4°C. The addition compound readily degrades above pH 6.0 to give the parent compound.[5] Solutions in dimethyl sulphoxide or dimethyl acetamide are stable for up to one year.[6] This formulation offers no advantages over the lyophilized preparation since it must be diluted prior to administration. It may also introduce difficulties with the extraction of plasticizer from PVC containers and administration sets.

4 Clinical Use

Type of cytotoxic: Inhibitor of DNA. Azacytidine causes hypomethylation of DNA which induces gene activation and expression and cell differentiation. This may be an underlying factor in its cytotoxic activity and also contributes to its carcinogenic and tumour-promoting properties. For a review of the clinical activity of azacytidine (see Glover *et al.*)[4]

Main indication: Acute myelogenous leukaemia.

Dosage: Up to 750 mg/m², usually 100 to 300 mg/m², daily × 5; every 8 hours × 15; 3 hour IV infusion every 8 hours × 5–7 days.

5 Preparation of Injection

Reconstitution: A 100 mg vial with 19.9 ml of water for injections gives a 5 mg/ml solution.

6 Destruction of Drug or Contaminated Articles

Incineration: 1000°C.

Chemical: No information.

Contact with skin: Wash with water.

References

1. Notari, R.E. and DeYoung, J.L. (1975). Kinetics and mechanisms of degradation of the antileukaemia agent 5-azacytidine in aqueous solutions. *J. Pharm. Sci.* **64**, 114–118.
2. Chan, K.K. *et al.* (1979). Azacytidine kinetics measured by high pressure liquid chromatography and ¹³C-NMR spectroscopy. *J. Pharm. Sci.* **68**, 807–812.
3. Cheung, Y-W. *et al.* (1984). Stability of azacytidine in infusion fluids. *Am. J. Hosp. Pharm.* **41**, 1156–1159.
4. Glover, A.B. *et al.* (1987). Azacytidine: 10 years later. *Cancer Treat. Rep.* **71**, 737–747.
5. Chatterji, D.C. and Gallelli, J.F. (1979). Stabilization of 5-azacytidine by nucleophilic addition of bisulphite ion. *J. Pharm. Sci.* **68**, 822–826.
6. Mojverian, P. and Repta, A.J. (1984). Development of an intravenous formulation for the unstable investigational cytotoxic nucleosides 5-azacytidine arabinoside (NSC 281272) and 5-azacytidine (NSC 102816). *J. Pharm. Pharmacol.* **36**, 728–733.

Prepared by M.G. Lee.

BLEOMYCIN

1 General Details

Approved name: Bleomycin, bleomycin sulphate.

Proprietary name: Bleomycin Lundbeck Injection.

Manufacturer or supplier: Lundbeck Ltd.

Presentation and formulation details: Cream-coloured freeze-dried plug of bleomycin sulphate equivalent to 15 IU bleomycin in a clear glass ampoule. Contains no excipients.

Storage and shelf-life of unopened container: Store at room temperature and protect from light.[1] Shelf-life is 3 years.

2 Chemistry

Type: Anti-tumour antibiotic.

Molecular structure: Glycopeptide. The drug consists of at least 10 components, the main ones being bleomycin A_2 and bleomycin B_2.[2]

Solubility in water: Very soluble.

3 Stability Profile

Physical and chemical stability

In physiological saline, stable at room temperature, protected from light for 28 days (data on file at company). Equally stable at 2 to 8°C.[2,3] Less stable in glucose.

Degradation pathways: No information available.

Physical: Stable in pH range 4–10.[4] Light may cause bleomycin to break down.[1]

Container compatibility: Early studies suggested that bleomycin components A_2 and B_2 may bind to PVC containers.[5,6] The stability of bleomycin in the following systems has been investigated by the manufacturer:

▼ 0.9% saline in an infusion bag (bleomycin 15 IU/100 ml).
▼ 5% glucose in an infusion bag (bleomycin 15 IU/100 ml).
▼ 0.9% saline in polypropylene syringes (bleomycin 60 IU/100 ml).

The stability of bleomycin A_2 and B_2 was evaluated after 28 days storage at room temperature in the dark. Bleomycin was found to be relatively stable in 0.9% saline with only 4% loss in infusion bags and 6% loss in plastic syringes. In contrast, a 54% loss occurred from the glucose solution in the infusion bag. It can be concluded that bleomycin is relatively stable in PVC containers and plastic syringes provided that the diluent is 0.9% saline.

Compatibility with other drugs: Compatible with water for injections, sodium chloride 0.9%, heparin sodium, vincristine, vinblastine, hydrocortisone sodium phosphate and phenytoin.[4]

Incompatible with ascorbic acid, hydrogen peroxide, any agents containing sulphydryl groups, amino acids, riboflavin, frusemide, aminophylline and diazepam.[4]

Stability in clinical practice

The solution, after reconstitution, is stable for at least seven days, protected from light and stored in the refrigerator. It is similarly stable after dilution in 0.9% saline. Drug diluted in 5% glucose or glucose/saline is liable to bind to PVC in an unpredictable manner[5] and should be restricted to a shelf-life of not more than 24 hours.

4 Clinical Use

Type of cytotoxic: Anti-tumour antibiotic.

Main indications: Squamous cell carcinoma. Hodgkin's disease and lymphomas, testicular teratoma, and malignant effusions of serous cavities.

Dosage: As single agent 15 to 30 IU twice or three times weekly up to a total of 100–500 IU, dependent on age and condition of patient; lower doses in combination therapy. For malignant effusions, use 60 IU in 100 ml physiological saline.

5 Preparation of Injection

Dilution: Dissolve dose in up to 5 ml water for injection or physiological saline. (1% lignocaine may be used if pain occurs at injection site. IM use only.)

Bolus administration: Inject slowly or via fast-running drip.

Infusion: Dilute in up to 200 ml physiological saline and administer slowly.

Gloves for handling: PVC or rubber.

Extravasation: Well tolerated by tissues so no treatment necessary.

6 Destruction of Drug or Contaminated Articles

Incineration: 1000°C.

Chemical: 10% sodium hydroxide or 1% potassium permanganate/24 hours.

Contact with skin: Wash with soap and water.

References

1. Douglas, K.T. (1983). Photoactivity of bleomycin. *Biomed. Pharmacother.* **37**, 191–193.
2. McEvoy, G.K. (ed.) (1985). *American Hospital Formulary service drug information.* American Society of Hospital Pharmacists, Bethesda, Maryland, USA.
3. Anon. (1981). *Outline guide for the use of cancer chemotherapeutic agents.* MD Anderson Hospital and Tumor Institute, University of Texas Cancer Center, Houston, Texas.
4. Dorr, R.T. *et al.* (1982). Bleomycin compatibility with selected intravenous medications. *J. Med.* **13**, 121–130.
5. Benvenuto, J.A. *et al.* (1981). Stability and compatibility of antitumor agents in glass and plastic containers. *Am. J. Hosp. Pharm.* **38**, 1914–1918.
6. Adams, J. *et al.* (1982). Instability of bleomycin in plastic containers. *Am. J. Hosp. Pharm.* **39**, 1636.

Prepared by R.J. Needle

CARBOPLATIN

1 General Details

Approved names: Carboplatin, JM8.

Proprietary names: Paraplatin.

Manufacturer or supplier: Bristol-Myers Pharmaceuticals Ltd and ER Squibb & Sons Ltd.

Presentation and formulation details: White freeze-dried powder in vials containing 50, 150 and 450 mg carboplatin. Formulation contains 50, 150 and 450 mg mannitol respectively/vial.

Storage and shelf-life of unopened container: 18 months at room temperature.[1]

2 Chemistry

Type: Platinum-containing complex.

Molecular structure: Cis-diammine (1,1-Cyclobutanedicarboxylato) platinum.

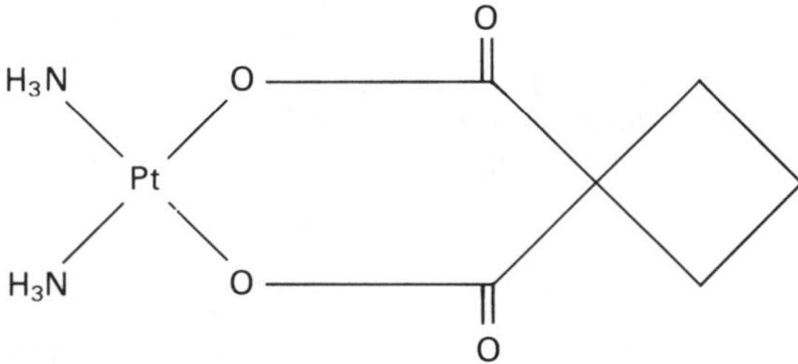

Molecular weight: 371.24.

Solubility in water: 18.6mg/ml.[2]

3 Stability Profile

Physical and chemical stability

Carboplatin is stable for 24 hours at room temperature in 5% glucose. It is less stable in 0.9% sodium chloride or glucose/saline injections.[3] Dilution of carboplatin with solutions containing chloride ions (eg 0.9% saline) leads to accelerated degradation, products including cisplatin.[3]

Degradation pathways: Carboplatin degrades by two simultaneous mechanisms:[5]

▼ hydrolytic reactions which give 'activated' platinum species
▼ nucleophilic substitution with chloride (and probably other nucleophiles) resulting in the replacement of the cyclo-butanecarboxylate ligands with chloride.

The overall rate of reaction can be described as:

$$K_{obs} = K_1 + K_2 (Cl^-)$$

Where K_{obs} = observed degradation constant
K_1 = hydrolytic rate constant
K_2 = chloride-dependent nucleophilic substitution rate constant.

Values of K_1 and K_2 at 25°C were 9.74×10^{-4} hr^{-1} and 3.14×10^{-3} hr^{-1}, respectively. Apparent first-order kinetics is obeyed.

The range of degradation products (some are intermediates) possibly include:

▼ monosubstitution with Cl$^-$;
▼ disubstitution with Cl$^-$ (cisplatin);
▼ monosubstitution with water;
▼ substitution with water and chloride ions.

The aquated 'intermediates' are likely to be the most toxic (but also the species with most anti-tumour activity). They can form various dimers, trimers and other oligomers in their own right.

Effect of temperature: The stability of carboplatin incubated at 4, 21 and 37°C in water, 0.9% saline or 5% glucose over 7 days is summarized in Table 1.[4]

Table 1: *The effect of temperature on stability of carboplatin (3.7 mg/ml) stored in different infusions*

Temp °C	Infusion					
	0.9% NaCl		Water		5% dextrose	
	T/5	t	T/5	t	T/5	t
4	24	322+31	32	403+84	40	506+94
21	22	291+44	32	409+82	44	539+44
37	9	116+6	14	223+21	16	244+16

Where t = half-life (hours); T/5 = 5% degradation (hours)

Stability is, therefore, not greatly influenced by temperatures between 4° and ambient.

Carboplatin is not especially light-sensitive.

Container compatibility: Carboplatin is compatible with PVC infusion containers[3] and plastic syringes.[6] In one study of the stability of carboplatin infusion (10 mg/ml) in water for injections there was no loss of carboplatin from pre-filled syringes stored at 4°C for five days.[4]

Compatibility with other drugs: Mixing carboplatin with any drug solution containing chloride ions (eg hydrochloride salts) leads to accelerated degradation.

Stability in clinical practice

If reconstituted in water for injections or 5% glucose as directed, it is stable for at least eight hours at room temperature or 24 hours if stored in a refrigerator.[1] Studies have indicated that the refrigerated solution in water for injections is stable for five days.[5] After dilution in 5% glucose, the infusion is stable for 24 hours in the refrigerator.[3]

It has been shown that, after 24 hours storage of solutions in 0.9% saline containing 1 mg/ml, less than 1% degradation to cisplatin has occurred.[7]

4 Clinical Use

Main indications: First or second line therapy of advanced ovarian carcinoma of epithelial origin and, small cell carcinoma of the lung.

Dosage and administration: Carboplatin should be administered intravenously. Recommended dosage in previously untreated adult patients with normal kidney function is 400 mg/m^2 as a single IV dose administered by a short-term (15 to 60 min) infusion.

Therapy should not be repeated until four weeks after the previous carboplatin course. Reduction of initial dosage by 20 to 25% is recommended for those patients with risk factors, eg prior myelosuppressive treatment.

Carboplatin should not be used in patients with severe pre-existing renal impairment (creatinine clearance at or below 20 ml/min).

5 Preparation of Injection

Reconstitution: Each vial is reconstituted with 15 ml of water for injections, 5% glucose injection or 0.9% sodium chloride injection to give a final concentration of 10 mg/ml.

Bolus administration: Must be further diluted.

Infusion: Dilute further, to as low as 500 μg/ml (1:20). Reconstituted solutions in 5% glucose or 0.9% sodium chloride for injection may be further diluted with the same vehicles originally used for reconstitution to concentrations as low as 0.5 mg/ml. Solutions originally reconstituted with water for injections may be further diluted with either of the other two fluids.

Gloves for handling: Rubber or polyethylene.

Extravasation: Non-irritant.

6 Destruction of Drug or Contaminated Articles

Incineration: 1000°C.

Chemical: None reported.

Contact with skin: Wash with water.

References

1. ABPI Data Sheet Compendium 1989/90. (1989). Datapharm Publications Ltd, London, pp. 253–255.
2. Harrap, K.R. (1986). Paraplatin preclinical development. In: *Abstracts of a symposium on paraplatin*, Imperial College, London, April 7th, 1986, pp. 3–7. Bristol-Myers Oncology.

3. Cheung, Y. *et al.* (1987). Stability of cisplatin, iproplatin, carboplatin and tetraplatin in commonly used infusion solutions. *Am. J. Hosp. Pharm.* **44**, 124–130.
4. Personal communication. (1988). Institute of Cancer Research, London. Unpublished Data.
5. Sewell, G.J. (1988). Personal communication.
6. Sewell, G.J. *et al.* (1987). The stability of Carboplatin in ambulatory continuous infusion regimens. *J. Clin. Pharm. Therap.* **12**, 427–432.
7. Perrone, R.K. *et al.* (1989). Extent of cisplatin formation in carboplatin admixtures. *Am. J. Hosp. Pharm.* **46**, 258–259.

Prepared by T. Root, assisted by K. Patel and G. Patel.

CARMUSTINE

1 General Details

Approved names: Carmustine, BCNU.

Proprietary names: Bicnu.

Manufacturer or supplier: Bristol-Myers Pharmaceuticals Ltd and ER Squibb & Sons Ltd.

Presentation and formulation details: White freeze-dried flaky powder in 30 ml capacity vial, containing 100 mg carmustine. Contains no excipients.

Storage and shelf-life of unopened container: Three years at 2 to 8°C, protect from light.

2 Chemistry

Type: nitrosourea.

Molecular structure: N,N'-bis(2-chloroethyl)-1-nitrosourea.

$$\text{ClCH}_2\text{CH}_2\text{N} \overset{\overset{\text{NO}}{|}}{-} \overset{\overset{\text{O}}{||}}{\text{C}} -\text{NHCH}_2\text{CH}_2\text{Cl}$$

Molecular weight: 214.04.

Melting point: 27°C.

Solubility: 4 mg/ml in water; 150 mg/ml in 95% ethanol.

3 Stability Profile

Physical and chemical stability

Carmustine is relatively unstable after reconstitution. Its stability depends on a number of factors. The most important chemical factor is pH.

Degradation pathways (in aqueous solution):[1] BCNU degrades to: 2 chloroethylamine hydrochloride + acetaldehyde + nitrogen + carbon dioxide. $Cl.CH_2\ CH_2\ NH_3\ HCl + CH_3CHO + N_2 + CO_2$).

Carmustine has a very low melting point (27°C according to the manufacturer, although another source quotes 30 to 32°C[2]). The drug, if melted, liquifies to become an oily film in the base of the vial. The physical change may also be associated with decomposition and such vials must be discarded. There is slow decomposition at room temperature. One report suggests 3% degradation in 36 days.[3]

The manufacturer indicates that the reconstituted injection decomposes by zero order kinetics. Thus, at ambient temperature, this report anticipated losses of 6% in three hours, whilst at 4°C losses of 4% in 24 hours are to be expected (the pH of the reconstituted injection is 5.6–6.0).

Studies[4,5] indicate that carmustine is most stable in aqueous buffered solutions between pH 3.5 and 5.0. In more acid conditions, there is a small increase in degradation rate whilst at pH above 4.8, degradation rates increase rapidly. For example at pH 5.0 (buffer) $t^{95\%}$ = 5 hours (24°C) or 60 hours (4°C), but at pH 7.3 (buffer) $t^{95\%}$ = 40 minutes (22°C) or 9 hours (4°C). Degradation may also be accelerated by buffering agents, especially phosphates.[1] The pH will rise during degradation in unbuffered medium, causing an acceleration in degradation rate with time. It has been suggested that because of the importance of pH, diluted solutions will be more stable in 5% glucose than in 0.9% sodium chloride.[5]

Effect of light: Fredriksson *et al.*[5] have shown that carmustine is relatively light sensitive. Under artificial laboratory conditions using a light cabinet, the reaction rates at various light intensities were reported. Samples were placed in covered Petri dishes, not accurately reflecting degradation rates in practice. The authors reported a value for $t^{10\%}$ of 2.9 hours at an intensity of 1000 lux (a relatively high light intensity). The light-induced degradation rate is reduced in a bulk solution packed in a glass or plastic infusion container. Degradation will also occur during passage of the infusion through the administration set. Unfortunately the data from this report cannot be used to predict the outcome of light-exposure in practice, but they do indicate the need to protect the drug from light-exposure during storage after reconstitution and dilution into infusions.

Effect of freezing: One report suggests that the drug is stable in infusions when in the frozen state,[5] but further studies are necessary to confirm this observation since evidence is somewhat conflicting.[6]

Container compatibility: Benvenuto *et al.*[7] indicated that infusions of carmustine in 5% glucose may be less stable in PVC than in glass containers. Some sorption to plastic containers (PVC

Viaflex) was indicated. Losses of the order of 10% after 0.5 to 1 hour and 35% after 4 hours were evident (drug concentration = 1.25 mg/ml in 5% glucose at pH 4.4). However, these tests were carried out in 50 ml bags; in 500 ml bags, the surface area to volume ratio is lower so absorption rates may be reduced.

More recent studies[4] suggest that carmustine interacts with PVC, EVA and polyurethane administration sets, whilst no sorption to polyethylene was apparent. Tests under simulated infusion conditions from glass bottles suggest that if 500 ml of drug (0.20 mg/ml) is infused over one hour, about 4.6% (4.6 mg) of the dose is lost by sorption, but over two hours 6.5% (6.5 mg) will be lost.

However, all of these tests were conducted at a drug concentration of about 0.2 mg/ml. No studies on the effect of drug concentration were reported. It is likely that the losses may be substantially reduced (as a proportion of the total dose) at higher drug concentrations.

The evidence, therefore, indicates that carmustine binds to some plastics, especially PVC, but the full clinical implications regarding dose delivery from an infusion are yet to be fully quantified. In practice, it may be relatively unimportant.

Stability in clinical practice

After reconstitution in the vial the injection can be stored for up to two days in the refrigerator. After dilution in 0.9% sodium chloride or 5% glucose in glass or polyethylene containers, the resulting infusion may be stored for up to two days in the refrigerator. If diluted in an infusion in a PVC container, it should not be stored, but used as soon as possible.

Carmustine is unstable after addition to any infusion containing sodium bicarbonate (due to alkaline pH).

4 Clinical Use

Type of cytotoxic: Nitrosourea, alkylating agent.

Main indications: Brain tumours. In combination therapy for multiple myeloma, Hodgkin's disease and other lymphomas.

Dosage: 200 mg/m^2 every six weeks as a single agent: lower doses when used in combination with other chemotherapeutic agents.

5 Preparation of Injection

Dilution: To each vial add 3 ml diluent (absolute ethanol), dissolve contents and then dilute with 27 ml water for injections. Resulting solution contains 3.3 mg in 1 ml of 10% ethanol. Dissolution may be faster if vial and diluent are allowed to come to room temperature.

Bolus administration: Not recommended but if essential, inject very slowly via the bolus site of a fast-running drip infusion: Dilute in 5% glucose (up to 500 ml), preferably in a glass or polyethylene (eg Polyfusor) container and administer over one to two hours as a slow infusion. Protect the contents from light by covering the infusion with a light-protecting overwrap if infused over two hours, or exposed to sunlight. Do not store in a PVC container but use immediately after preparation. Non-PVC containing sets (eg Sureset, Avon Medical) are recommended.

Gloves for handling: Rubber gloves are recommended. Carmustine will penetrate all types – two layers recommended.[8]

Extravasation: Damaging; the antidote is 8.4% sodium bicarbonate injection.

6 Destruction of Drug or Contaminated Articles

Incineration: 800°C.

Chemical: Sodium bicarbonate solution/24 to 48 hours.

Contact with skin: Wash with copious amounts of water. In some cases of local irritancy apply sodium bicarbonate solution.

References

1. Montgomery, J.A. *et al.* (1967). The modes of decomposition of 1.3-bis (2-chloro-ethyl)-1-nitrosourea and related compounds. *J. Med. Chem.* **10**, 668–674.
2. Trissel, L.A. (1988). *Handbook of injectable drugs*, 5th edn, American Society of Hospital Pharmacists, Bethesda, Maryland, USA.
3. Kleinman, L.M. *et al.* (1976). Investigational drug information. *Drug Intell. Clin. Pharm.* **10**, 48–49.
4. Lasker, P.A. and Ayres, J.W. (1977). Degradation of carmustine in aqueous media. *J. Pharm. Sci.* **66**, 1073–1076.
5. Fredriksson, K. *et al.* (1986). Stability of carmustine-kinetics and compatibility during administration. *Acta Pharm.* **23**, 115–124.
6. Bosanquet, A.G. (1985). Stability of solutions of antineoplastic agents during preparation and storage for *in vitro* assays. General considerations and nitrosoureas and alkylating agents. *Cancer Chemother. Pharmacol.* **14**, 83–95.
7. Benvenuto, J.A. *et al.* (1981). Stability and compatibility of antitumour agents in glass and plastic containers. *Am. J. Hosp. Pharm.* **38**, 1914–1918.
8. Thomas, P.H. and Fenton-May, V. (1987). Protection offered by various gloves to carmustine exposure. *Pharm. J.* **238**, 775–777.

Prepared by M.C. Allwood

CISPLATIN

1 General Details

Approved names: Cisplatin, cis DDP.

Proprietary names: Cisplatin.

Manufacturers or suppliers: David Bull Laboratories Ltd (DBL), Farmitalia Carlo Erba Ltd, Lederle Laboratories Ltd. DBL, Lederle, and Farmitalia supply cisplatin as both solution and powder.

The powder is either freeze-dried or lyophilized (see Table 1). The solution is clear, practically colourless and is supplied in amber glass vials. The pH of both is usually between 3.5 and 5.5.

Presentation and formulation details: Some preparations contain mannitol to aid diuresis and renal clearance of cisplatin. Sodium chloride is added to improve chemical stability (*see* Stability Profile for further information).

Storage and shelf-life of unopened container: Both the powder and the solution preparations should be stored at controlled room temperature (15 to 30°C) and protected from direct bright sunlight. Protection from normal room fluorescent light is also recommended.[9] Unopened vials of the drug are stable for 2 to 3 years (depending on the manufacturer).

2 Chemistry

Type: Platinum-containing complex.

Molecular structure: The platinum atom is surrounded in a plane by two chloride atoms and 2 ammonia molecules, in the cis position, platinum diammino dichloride.

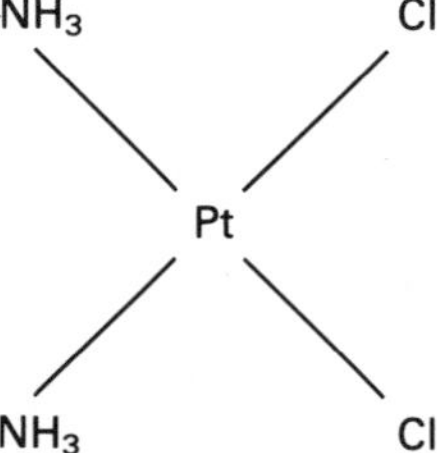

Molecular weight: 300.1.

Solubility: 1 mg/1 ml in water; 1 g in 42 ml of dimethyl formamide.

3 Stability Profile

Physical and chemical stability

Cisplatin is unstable in an aqueous vehicle unless chloride ions are present. For example, losses of 30 to 35% in four hours, or 70 to 80% in 24 hours at 25°C have been reported.[1] The minimum concentration of sodium chloride providing an acceptable level of stability is about 0.3% w/v[2] (weight by volume).

Table 1: *Forms of cisplatin available*

Manufacturer	Form	Amount of cisplatin	Strength of solution	Strength of solution after reconstitution	Mannitol per ml of solution	NaCl per ml of solution
DBL	solution	10 mg	1 mg/ml		10 mg	9 mg
	solution	50 mg	1 mg/ml		10 mg	9 mg
	solution	100 mg	1 mg/ml		10 mg	9 mg
	powder	10 mg				
	powder	50 mg				
Farmitalia	solution	10 mg	0.5 mg/ml		–	9 mg
	solution	50 mg	0.5 mg/ml		–	9 mg
	freeze-dried powder	10 mg		1 mg/ml	30 mg	4.5 mg
	powder	50 mg		1 mg/ml	30 mg	4.5 mg
Lederle	solution	10 mg	1 mg/ml		10 mg	12 mg
	solution	25 mg	1 mg/ml		10 mg	12 mg
	solution	50 mg	1 mg/ml		10 mg	12 mg
	lyophilized powder	10 mg		1 mg/ml	10 mg	9 mg
	lyophilized powder	50 mg		1 mg/ml	10 mg	9 mg

Solutions of cisplatin in 0.9% sodium chloride are relatively stable for at least 24 hours at ambient temperatures. It should be noted that an equilibrium will be established between cisplatin and chloride ions in solution (see below). In 0.9% sodium chloride, approximately 97% cisplatin will be present at equilibrium.[1,3] This level of degradation does not seriously compromise therapeutic efficacy or toxicity profiles. Other studies have indicated that dilutions of cisplatin injection in 0.9% sodium chloride are chemically stable (< 5% degradation) for four days at 4°C, two days at 25°C or 30 days at −15°C.[4] The pH does not appear to be an important factor in cisplatin injection stability after dilution in recommended infusion fluids. Cisplatin is also stable in 0.9% sodium chloride in the presence of magnesium sulphate and potassium chloride for up to 24 hours.[9]

Degradation pathways: Cisplatin undergoes nucleophilic displacement of the chloride ligand by water in aqueous media[3,5] (*see* Figure 1). It is believed that the major route of decomposition involves the displacement of one chloride ion. The loss of the second chloride ion may not contribute substantially to the overall decomposition rate. The reaction is reversible. When enough liberated chloride ions accumulate in the medium, the reaction reaches an equilibrium. The equilibrium drug concentration depends on the concentration of chloride ions present. (Cisplatin can re-form in decomposed drug solutions with the addition of sufficient amounts of chloride.)

The reactions can be described by first order kinetics, dependent principally on chloride ion concentration. Only the first reaction is of practical significance.[1,3]

Effect of light: Cisplatin is relatively sensitive to daylight, but reports confirm that the drug is not adversely affected by normal room lighting after dilution in 0.9% sodium chloride[1,9] (*see* Table 2).

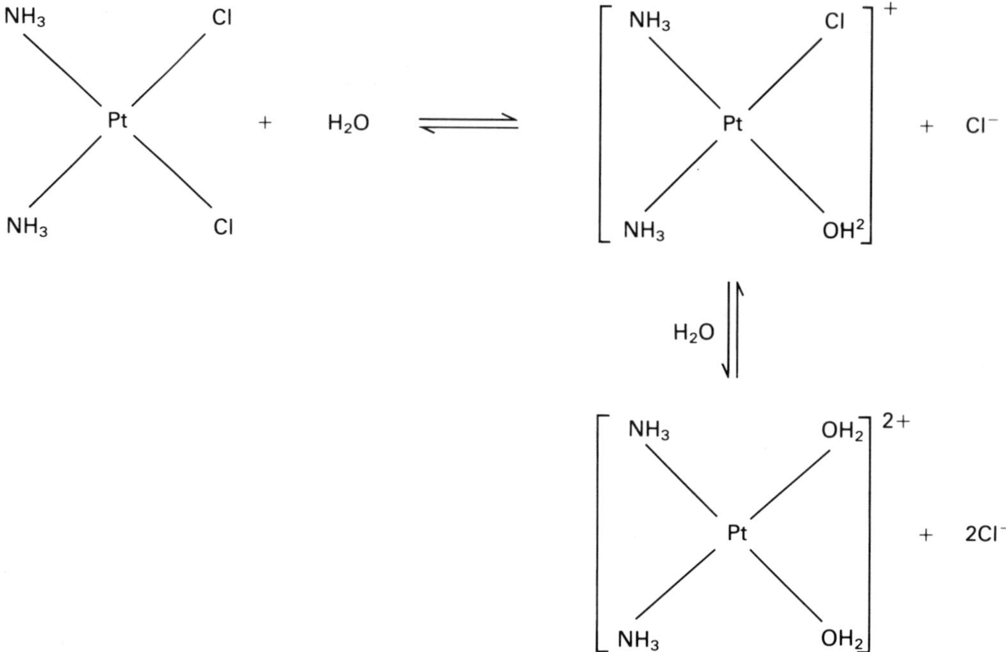

Figure 1: *Degradation pathways proposed for cisplatin*

Table 2: *Stability of cisplatin injection in 0.9% sodium chloride*

Time	Storage Condition 20°C			
	Viaflex container/bag		Glass bottle	
	exposed to light % cisplatin	protected from light % cisplatin	exposed to light % cisplatin	protected from light % cisplatin
0 day	100.0 pH 4.60	100.0 pH 4.90	100.0 pH 4.90	100.0 pH 4.95
4 days	89.2 + 0.2* pH 5.90	100.0 + 0.1 pH 4.87	83.8 + 0.2 pH 6.76	99.5 + 0.1 pH 5.35
7 days	85.9 + 0.2 pH: not recorded	100.5 + 0.3	79.0 + 0.1	100.2 + 0.1
14 days	77.2 + 0.2 pH 6.85	99.8 + 0.1 pH 4.70	70.1 + 0.2 pH 7.23	99.5 + 0.3 pH 4.86

* The figures represent the mean + standard deviation.

The solutions at the concentration of 150 mg cisplatin per 1000 ml 0.9% sodium chloride injection remained clear, colourless and free from particulate matter during the testing period.

Effect of temperature: Temperature appears to have little influence on the stability of cisplatin after dilution. However, because of limited solubility of cisplatin, especially in chloride-containing solutions, the cooling of diluted solutions can lead to precipitation. Studies have also shown that precipitates of cisplatin may be redissolved without further degradation by placing in a water bath heated to 70°C for four hours.[9] Concentrations of 1 mg/ml remain in solution at ambient temperature, while refrigeration can lead to precipitation within one hour.[4,6] Solutions stored in a refrigerator should contain NMT 0.6 mg/ml if stored for 24 hours or NMT 0.5 mg/ml if stored for 24 to 72 hours.[7] Further studies have shown that solutions containing 0.05 to 0.2 mg/ml remain potent for four days at 4°C.[4]

Container compatibility: Cisplatin diluted in 0.9% sodium chloride is stable in glass or PVC containers.[2,4] Cisplatin reacts with aluminium and care should be taken to avoid contact of injections with metal items containing aluminium. Stainless steel is compatible.[8]

Compatibility with other drugs: Cisplatin injection is compatible with mannitol and magnesium sulphate injection.[4] However, it has been suggested that mannitol–cisplatin complexes may form if diluted mixtures are stored for several days.[5] Mannitol should therefore be added immediately before administration if 'diuresis' doses are required.

Stability in clinical practice

Reconstituted or diluted cisplatin injections are stable, if diluted in 0.9% sodium chloride, for 20 hours at 25°C but will precipitate on refrigeration.[7] In practice, the appropriate dose should be diluted in 2 L 0.9% sodium chloride infusion, giving concentrations in the range 0.1 to 0.2 mg/ml. At such concentrations precipitation will not occur on refrigeration. Such dilute infusions are stable for four days at 4°C in PVC containers.[4]

4 Clinical Use

Type of cytotoxic: platinum-containing complex. The exact mechanism of action has not been determined conclusively but the drug has biochemical properties similar to those of alkylating agents.

Main indications: Cisplatin is used for many indications and in varying doses, commonly 20–100 mg/m^2.

5 Preparation of Injection

Reconstitution: Cisplatin powder should be dissolved in the diluent provided or water for injections to give 0.5 or 1 mg/ml, as directed (*see* Table 1). The manufacturers recommend that cisplatin solution is added to 2 L of 0.9% sodium chloride solution although, at The Royal Marsden Hospital, doses of up to 100 mg/m^2 cisplatin are added to as little as 250 ml of 0.9% sodium chloride solution. Larger doses would be added to 500 ml to 1000 ml. The resulting infusion bag should be protected from light and stored at room temperature.

Bolus administration: Must not be used.

Infusion: The manufacturers recommend that cisplatin solution be infused over six to eight hours although at The Royal Marsden Hospital a dose of less than 100 mg in 250 ml 0.9% sodium chloride is infused over 30 minutes. Larger doses are often given over one to two hours or longer if renal function is particularly poor. Pre- and post-hydration are essential to induce diuresis during and after the cisplatin infusion. This is to ensure adequate renal clearance of cisplatin and varies according to the dose.

Below are The Royal Marsden Hospital procedures for pre- and post-hydration, for varying doses of cisplatin:

▼ 20 mg/m²: Pre-hydrate with 1 L 0.9% sodium chloride infusion over six hours. Give 1 L 4% glucose/0.18% sodium chloride +20 mmol KCl every eight hours for 24 hours after cisplatin treatment.

▼ 50 mg/m²: Pre-hydrate with I L 0.9% sodium chloride infusion over six hours followed by 100 ml 20% mannitol over 30 minutes. After cisplatin, give 1 L 0.9% sodium chloride infusion + 20 mmol KCl every eight hours for 24 hours.

▼ 100 mg/m²: Pre-hydrate with I L 0.9% sodium chloride infusion + 20 mmol KCl every eight hours × 3 followed by 200 ml mannitol 20% over 30 minutes. After cisplatin give I L 0.9% sodium chloride + 20 mmol KCl over 4 hours and then 0.9% sodium chloride + 20 mmol KCl every 8 hours × 3.

Gloves for handling: Rubber gloves should be used.

Extravasation: Non-irritant.

6 Destruction of Drug or Contaminated Articles

Incineration: 800°C.

Chemical: Dilute in large volume of water, allow to stand for 48 hours.

Contact with skin: Wash with copious amounts of water. Apply a cream if transient stinging is experienced. (NB: Some individuals are sensitive to platinum and a skin reaction may occur.)

References

1. Hincal, A.A. *et al.* (1979). Cisplatin stability in aqueous parenteral vehicles. *J. Parenteral Drug. Assoc.* **33**, 107–116.
2. Cheung, Y.H. *et al.* (1987). Stability of cisplatin, iproplatin, carboplatin and tetraplatin in commonly used intravenous solutions. *Am. J. Hosp. Pharm.* **44**, 124–130.
3. Le Rey, R.H. (1970). Some quantitative data on cis-dichlorodiammineplatinum (II) species in solution. *Cancer Treat. Rep.* **63**, 231–233.
4. La Follette, J.M. *et al.* (1985). Stability of cisplatin admixtures in polyvinyl chloride bags. *Am. J. Hosp. Pharm.* **42**, 2652.

5. Trissel, L.A. (1988). *Handbook of injectable drugs*. 5th edn, American Society of Hospital Pharmacists, Bethesda, Maryland, USA.
6. Green, R.F. *et al.* (1979). Stability of cisplatin in aqueous solution. *Am. J. Hosp. Pharm.* **36**, 38–43.
7. ABPI Data Sheet Compendium 1989/90. (1989). Datapharm Publications Ltd, London, pp. 462–464, 755–757.
8. Bohart, R.D. and Ogawa, G. (1979). An observation on the stability of Cis-dichlorodiammineplatinum (II): A caution regarding its administration. *Cancer Treat. Rep.* **63**, 2117–2118.
9. Personal communications, DBL Ltd. Unpublished Data.

Prepared by T. Root and K. Patel.

CYCLOPHOSPHAMIDE

1 General Details

Approved names: Cyclophosphamide, cyclophospham.

Proprietary names: Endoxana, cyclophosphamide.

Manufacturers or suppliers: Farmitalia Carlo Erba Ltd, Degussa Pharmaceuticals Ltd.

Presentation and formulation details: Sterile, white powder in vials containing: 107 mg, 214 mg, 535 mg or 1069 mg of cyclophosphamide equivalent to 100 mg, 200 mg, 500 mg or 1000 mg respectively, of anhydrous cyclophosphamide. Sodium chloride is also present to render the solution isotonic after reconstitution with the recommended amount of water for injections.[1,2]

Storage and shelf-life of unopened container: Cyclophosphamide should be stored in a cool place (below 25°C), away from heat sources. It should be protected from light and is stable in the vial for five years.[1,2]

2 Chemistry

Type: Cyclophosphamide is a cytotoxic which is converted in the body to an active alkylating agent with properties similar to those of mustine.[3]

Molecular structure: Cyclophosphamide (Farmitalia Carlo Erba) contains 2-[bis (2 chloroethyl) amino]-perhydro-1,3,2 oxazophosphorine-2-oxide monohydrate.

$$\left[\text{O}\diagdown \underset{\underset{\text{NH}}{|}}{\overset{\diagup\text{O}}{\text{P}}} \diagdown \text{N(CH}_2\cdot\text{CH}_2\cdot\text{Cl)}_2 \right] \quad \text{H}_2\text{O}$$

Molecular weight: 279.1.

Melting point: 49.5 to 53°C.[3] Endoxana (Degussa Pharmaceuticals) contains the anhydrous salt.

Molecular weight: 261.08.

Melting point: 41 to 45°C.[4]

Solubility: Cyclophosphamide is soluble 1 in 25 parts of water and 0.9% sodium chloride and 1 in 1 of alcohol.[3,5]

3 Stability Profile

The manufacturer recommends that the reconstituted solution (20 mg/ml) is used within eight hours when stored at room temperature (25°C).[1] A review of the literature reveals that cyclophosphamide may be chemically stable for longer periods if stored at 4°C.

Physical and chemical stability

The loss of cyclophosphamide monohydrate from aqueous solution results from hydrolysis, loss of a chloride ion, or both.[6–9] Degradation follows first order kinetics and is accompanied by a slight downward shift in pH which does not appear to affect the kinetics of drug loss.[10] During degradation the solution remains colourless.[10] Increase in temperature accelerates the rate of breakdown, as can the presence of benzyl alcohol.[10]

Effect of pH: Hirata *et al.*[6] showed that the rate constant for drug loss at 75°C was independent of pH (pH 2 to 10).
Outside these limits acidic and basic catalysis was observed. In solutions between pH 2 and pH 14 cyclophosphamide degrades via a bicyclic compound, and a number of secondary intermediates, to give N-(2-hydroxyethyl)-N′-(3-hydroxypropyl) ethylenediamine.[7,11,12] The mechanism for hydrolysis of cyclophosphamide proposed by Chakrabarti and Friedman[11] is shown in Figure 1.

Under more acidic conditions (pH ≤ 1) cyclophosphamide degrades via a different mechanism to yield bis (2-chloroethyl) amine and 3-aminopropan-1-ol.[6,12]

Effect of light: There are no published data which have systematically compared photodegradation of cyclophosphamide with degradation in identical solutions stored in the dark. Two studies have examined degradation in solutions of cyclophosphamide which were not protected from light. Gallelli[13] observed that cyclophosphamide, 4 mg/ml in 0.9% sodium chloride, stored in glass vials, exhibited 3.5% decomposition over a period of 24 hours at room temperature. Benvenuto *et al.*[14] observed that solutions of cyclophosphamide, 6.6 mg/ml in 5% glucose in both PVC and glass, were stable (< 10% degradation) for 24 hours at room temperature. From these data it is difficult to draw conclusions about the effect of light on the stability of cyclophosphamide.

Effect of temperature: If heated above 32°C cyclophosphamide may decompose to a damp-looking gel which should not be used.[1] The effect of briefly heating cyclophosphamide has been studied. Heating a solution containing 21 mg/ml of cyclophosphamide to 50 or 60°C for 15 minutes resulted in a negligible loss of potency.[15] However, heating to 70 or 80°C for 15 minutes resulted in approximately 10 and 23% decomposition respectively.[15] For this reason, the use of heat to speed up dissolution of cyclophosphamide is not recommended since decomposition may result.[15]

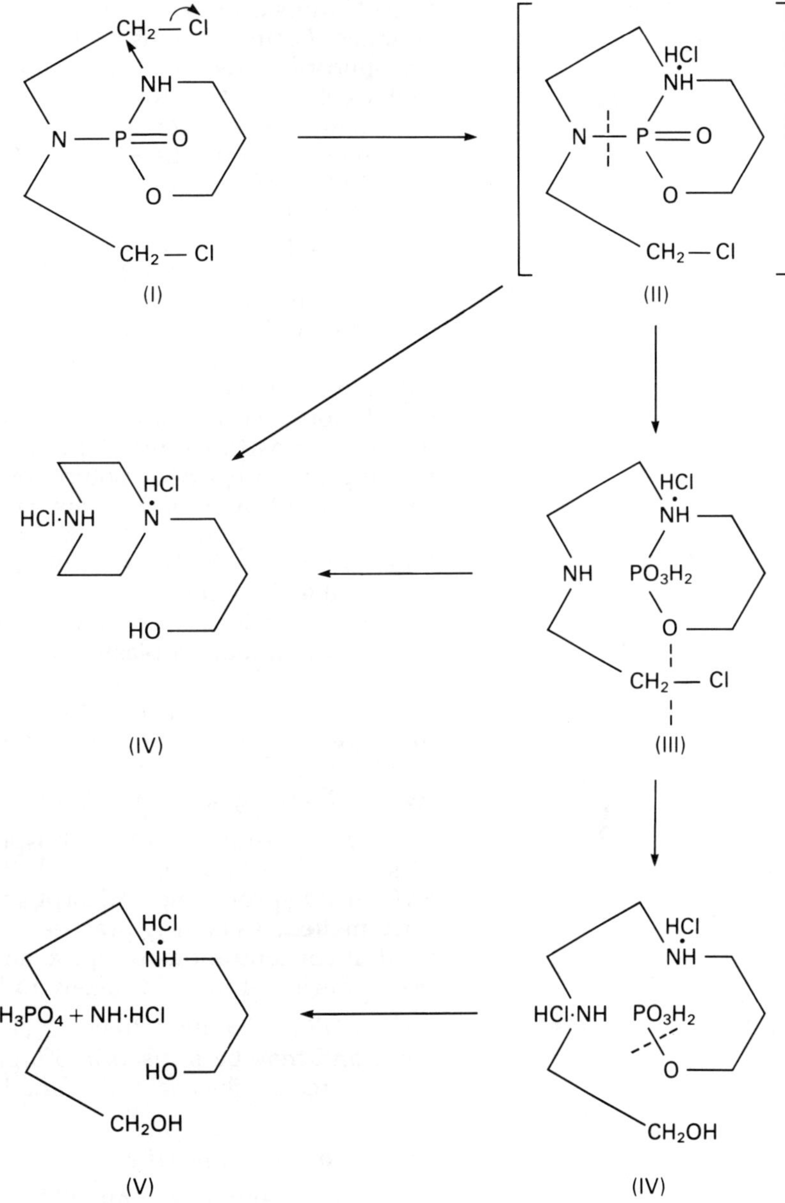

Figure 1: *Degradation of cyclophosphamide*[11]

Brook *et al.*[10] observed a 2% loss in potency in a solution of cyclophosphamide, 20 mg/ml, in glass vials, after four days storage at room temperature (24 to 27°C) and an 8% loss after 17 weeks at 4°C. The rates constants for drug loss recorded in that study were not significantly different for solutions reconstituted with water for injections, glucose 5% or glucose/saline admixtures.

Kirk *et al.*[16] studied the stability of cyclophosphamide in glass ampoules, polypropylene syringes and PVC infusion containers. In PVC infusion bags (Viaflex, Baxter), polypropylene syringes (Becton Dickinson, Plastipak), and glass ampoules, cyclophosphamide showed no appreciable degradation after four weeks at 4°C. After 19 weeks at 4°C, 5.7% and 8% degradation was observed in solutions stored in syringes and minibags respectively.

The effect of freezing cyclophosphamide was also investigated by Kirk *et al.*[16] Results showed that in syringes, PVC minibags or glass ampoules, no appreciable degradation occurred after four weeks storage at −20°C. After 19 weeks, 4% and 8% degradation was observed in syringes and infusion bags respectively. However, two problems were encountered with freezing cyclophosphamide. Firstly, at higher concentrations (20 mg/ml) precipitation occurred during thawing. Although dissolution occurred after vigorous shaking, the possibility of injecting particles into the patient arises. Secondly, during freezing the integrity of polypropylene syringes was compromised by a marked contraction of the plungers allowing seepage of fluid past the plunger and on to the inner surface of the barrel. Although this probably represents a negligible drug loss, the potential risk of microbial contamination is unacceptable. Therefore, freezing of cyclophosphamide in plastic syringes is not recommended.

The effect of thawing cyclophosphamide in a microwave has also been investigated.[16] Results indicated that during microwave thawing uneven distribution of energy may occur and lead to overheating and consequent degradation. For this reason, thawing solutions in a microwave is not recommended.

Container compatibility: Cyclophosphamide is compatible with glass, PVC and polypropylene.[16] It is not adsorbed on to either PVC or polypropylene. Adsorption on to glass has not been documented. In clinical practice, when cyclophosphamide is used at concentrations of approximately 20 mg/ml, adsorptive losses during storage are likely to be negligible.[16]

Compatibility with other drugs: Cyclophosphamide is compatible with, and may be infused in 5% glucose, 0.9% sodium chloride or mixtures of glucose and saline.[17]

Stability in clinical practice

Cyclophosphamide is compatible with glass, PVC and polypropylene containers and appears to be chemically stable for at least 28 days when stored at 4°C.[16] Solutions of cyclophosphamide should not be frozen.

4 Clinical Use

Type of cytotoxic: Cyclophosphamide is a pro-drug which requires liver metabolism before becoming cytotoxic.

Main indications: It is used both as a single agent and in combination chemotherapy for a wide range of neoplastic diseases, including Burkitt's lymphoma, Hodgkin's lymphoma, acute and chronic leukaemia and multiple myeloma. Cyclophosphamide is also used in some solid tumours including carcinoma of the breast, cervix, lung and ovary; neuroblastoma, retinoblastoma and sarcomas.[1,2]

Dosage and administration: The dose, route and frequency of administration should be determined by the tumour type, tumour stage, the general condition of the patient and whether other chemotherapy or radiation is to be administered concurrently. The following sample regimens may serve as guides.

▼ Low dose: 80 to 240 mg/m^2 (2 to 6 mg/kg) as a single dose intravenously each week or as divided doses orally.
▼ Medium dose: 400 to 600 mg/m^2 (10 to 15 mg/kg) as a single dose intravenously each week.
▼ High dose: 800 to 1600 mg/m^2 (20 to 40 mg/kg) as a single dose at 10 to 20 day intervals.
▼ Very high dose: 60 to 80 mg/kg as a single dose intravenously at three to four week intervals.

It is recommended that the dose of cyclophosphamide is reduced when it is given in combination with other cytotoxic agents or radiotherapy, and in patients with bone marrow depression.[1,2]

Cyclophosphamide is metabolized to a compound (acrolein) which is toxic to the bladder. During treatment, a large urine output ($\geq$ 100 ml/hr) should be maintained to avoid haemorrhagic cystitis.[1] In addition, intravenous or oral mesna may be given concurrently.[18]

5 Preparation of Injection

Reconstitution: The contents of a vial are reconstituted with Water for Injections (5 ml per 100 mg of anhydrous cyclophosphamide). After addition of the diluent and vigorous shaking the contents of the vial will dissolve to produce a solution of 20 mg/ml. Formation of a solution may be delayed because of the slow dissolution rate of cyclophosphamide in aqueous media. The pH of an aqueous solution is between 4.5 and 5.5.[1] Water for injections preserved with benzyl alcohol should not be used for preparation.[10,19]

Bolus administration: Cyclophosphamide is usually given directly into a vein, over two or three minutes, or directly into the tubing of a fast running intravenous infusion. Cyclophosphamide injection may also be given intraperitoneally or intrapleurally but these routes offer no therapeutic advantage over the intravenous route.[1,2] Cyclophosphamide has also been given intra-arterially and by local perfusion. Cyclophosphamide may also be given orally as 50 mg tablets.[1] An elixir may be prepared by dissolving the contents of the dry powder vial in Aromatic Elixir USP shortly before administration.[3]

Infusion: High doses of cyclophosphamide may be added to an infusion of 5% glucose, 0.9% sodium chloride or glucose/saline and infused over 1 to 2 hours. Both prolonged intermittent and continuous infusion of cyclophosphamide have been studied.[20–24] In a phase I study, patients received 300 mg/m²/day to 750 mg/m²/day by continuous infusion over 72 hours.[22] Another study employed a five day continuous infusion at a rate of 400 mg/m²/day.[20] Protracted infusion of cyclophosphamide has been reported by Lokich *et al.*[24] at doses of 50 to 100 mg/m²/day for periods of 28 days or more.

Gloves for handling: Rubber gloves are recommended.

Extravasation: Cyclophosphamide is non-irritant but care should be taken that extravasation does not take place. However, should it occur, no specific measures need to be taken because the drug has to be activated in the liver before it becomes cytotoxic.

6 Destruction of Drug or Contaminated Articles

Incineration: 900°C.[4,25]

Chemical: 0.2 M potassium hydroxide in methanol solution/one hour or a 5% NaOCl solution/24 hours.[4,25]

Contact with skin: Wash with water, or soap and water. If the eyes are contaminated immediate irrigation with 0.9% sodium chloride should be carried out.[1,2]

References

1. Data sheet: cyclophosphamide, Degussa Pharmaceuticals.
2. ABPI Data Sheet Compendium 1989/1990. (1989). Datapharm Publications Ltd, London pp. 464–465.
3. Anon. (1989). *The extra pharmacopoeia*, 29th edn, Reynolds J.E.F. (ed.), Pharmaceutical Press, London, pp. 610–614.
4. Personal communication, Degussa Pharmaceuticals. Unpublished information.
5. Dorr, R.T. and Fritz, W.L. (1980). Cancer chemotherapy handbook, Elsevier, Amsterdam, p. 342.
6. Hirata, M. *et al.* (1967). Studies on cyclophosphamide. Part 1. Chemical determination and degradation kinetics in aqueous media. *Shionogi Kenkyusho Nempo*, **17**, 107–113.
7. Friedman, O.M. (1967). Recent biological and chemical studies of cyclophosphamide (NSC 26271). *Cancer Chemother. Rep.* **51**, 327–333.
8. Arnold, H. and Klose, H. (1961). Die hydrolyse hexacyclisher N-lostphosphamidester in gepufferten system. *Arzneimittel-Forsch*, **11**, 159–163.
9. Friedman, O.M. (1965). Studies on the hydrolysis of cyclophosphamide. I. Identification of N-(2-hydroxyethyl)-N'-(3-hydroxypropyl) ethylenediammine as the main product. *J. Am. Chem. Soc.* **87**, 4978–4979.

10. Brooke, D. *et al.* (1973). Chemical stability of cyclophosphamide in parenteral solutions. *Am. J. Hosp. Pharm.* **30**, 134–137.
11. Chakrabarti, J.K. and Friedman, O.M. (1973). Studies on the hydrolysis of cyclophosphamide. II. Isolation and characterisation of intermediate hydrolytic products.(I). *J. Heterocyclic Chemistry*, **10**, 55–58.
12. Zon, G. *et al.* (1977). High resolution nuclear magnetic resonance investigations of the chemical stability of cyclophosphamide and related phosphoramidic compounds. *J. Am. Chem. Soc.* **99(17)**, 5785–5795.
13. Gallelli, J.F. (1967). Stability studies of drugs used in intravenous solutions; Part one. *Am. J. Hosp. Pharm.* **24**, 425–433.
14. Benvenuto, J.A. *et al.* (1981). Stability and compatibility of antitumour agents in glass and plastic containers. *Am. J. Hosp. Pharm.* **38**, 1914–1918.
15. Brooke, D. *et al.* (1975). Effect of briefly heating cyclophosphamide solutions. *Am. J. Hosp. Pharm.* **32**, 44–45.
16. Kirk, B. *et al.* (1984). Chemical stability of cyclophosphamide injection. The effect of low temperature storage and microwave thawing. *Brit. J. Parenteral Therapy.* 90–97.
17. Trissel, L.A. (1988). *Handbook of injectable drugs*, 5th edn, American Society of Hospital Pharmacists, Bethesda, Maryland, USA.
18. ABPI Data Sheet Compendium 1989/1990. (1989). Datapharm Publications Ltd, London pp. 219–220.
19. D'Arcy, P.F. (1983). Handling anticancer drugs. *Drug Intell. Clin. Pharm.* **17**, 532–538.
20. Tchekmedyian, N.S. *et al.* (1986). Phase I clinical and pharmacokinetic study of cyclophosphamide administered by 5 day continuous intravenous infusion. *Cancer Chemother. Rep.* **18(1)**, 33–38.
21. Solidoro, A. *et al.* (1981). Intermittent continuous IV infusion of high dose cyclophosphamide for remission induction in acute lymphocytic leukaemia. *Cancer Treat. Rep.* **65**, 213–218.
22. Bedikian, A.Y. and Bodey, G.P. (1983). Phase I study of cyclophosphamide (NSC 26271) by 72-hour continuous intravenous infusion. *Am. J. Clin. Oncol.* **6**, 365–368.
23. Smith, D.B. *et al.* (1986). A phase II study of cyclophosphamide as a 24-hour infusion in advanced non small cell lung cancer. *Eur. J. Cancer Clin. Oncol.* **22**, 435–437.
24. Lokich, J.J. and Botha, A. (1984). Phase I study of continuous infusion cyclophosphamide for protracted duration: A preliminary report. *Cancer Drug Deliv.* **1**, 329–332.
25. Personal communication with Farmitalia Carlo Erba Ltd.

Prepared by M.J. Wood.

CYTARABINE

1 General Details

Approved names: Cytarabine, arabinosylcytosine, ara-C, cytosine, arabinoside.

Proprietary names: Alexan, Alexan 100, Cytosar.

Manufacturers or suppliers: Pfizer Ltd, Upjohn Ltd, David Bull Laboratories Ltd (DBL).

Presentation and formulation details:
▼ Alexan: 2 ml and 5 ml ampoules of an isotonic solution of cytarabine 20 mg/ml.
▼ Alexan 100: 1 ml and 10 ml ampoules of a hypertonic solution of cytarabine 100 mg/ml.

All solutions of Alexan and Alexan 100 are preservative free.[1]

▼ Cytosar: An off-white freeze-dried cake of 100 mg or 500 mg cytarabine in a rubber capped vial with a vial of solvent (water for injections containing 0.9% benzyl alcohol). Either sodium hydroxide or hydrochloric acid can be added to adjust the pH of the solution to approximately 5 when reconstituted as instructed.[2]
▼ Cytarabine: Vials containing 100 mg, 500 mg and 1000 mg with preserved diluent supplied.[3]

Storage and shelf-life of unopened container: Alexan solution in unopened ampoules is stable for three years from the date of manufacture when stored below 15°C.[1,4] Vials of Cytosar and cytarabine (DBL) are stable for three years from the date of manufacture when stored at room temperature.[3,5]

2 Chemistry

Type: Cytarabine is a pyrimidine nucleoside analogue that kills cells undergoing DNA synthesis. Its actions are specific for the S phase of the cell cycle.[6]

Molecular structure: 4-Amino-1-β-D arabinofuranosylpyrimidin-2-(1H)-one.

NH_2

N

O

N

$HOCH_2$ O

HO

OH

Molecular weight: 243.2.

Solubility: Cytarabine is soluble 1 in 10 parts of water and 1 in 1000 of alcohol.[6]

3 Stability Profile

Physical and chemical stability

The manufacturer states that ampoules of Alexan should be discarded within 24 hours of opening. Alexan and Alexan 100 are stable for at least 24 hours following dilution with 0.9% sodium chloride or 5% glucose infusion.[1] After reconstitution with unpreserved diluents the manufacturers recommend that Cytosar should be discarded immediately and not stored.[2] When reconstituted with the accompanying diluent solutions should be stored at room temperature and discarded within 48 hours.[2] A review of the literature reveals that cytarabine may be chemically stable for longer periods.

In aqueous buffered solution cytarabine is broken down by hydrolytic deamination to uracil arabinoside.[7] Breakdown is more rapid under alkaline than acid conditions.

Effect of pH: Cytarabine is most stable in the neutral pH region and has been calculated to retain 90% potency for six and a half months in 0.06 M phosphate buffer, pH 6.9, at 25°C. The rate of degradation of cytarabine in alkaline solution is approximately 10 times as great as in acidic solution.[8]

In aqueous buffered solutions cytarabine (I) has been shown to undergo hydrolytic deamination to form the inactive nucleoside arabinosyluracil (II). In the acid to neutral region, pH 0 to 7.8, I undergoes deamination to yield II via an intermediate, which is formed in maximum yield at pH 2 to 3, and is not formed in detectable yields at pH 5.5 to 7.8. The observed rate constant for the loss of I in the absence of buffer catalysis was found to pass through a maximum value at approximately pH 2.8. The proposed mechanism for the acid-catalysed degradation of cytarabine in aqueous solution, from Notari *et al.*[8] is shown in Figure 1.

The loss of I in alkaline solution is not accompanied by a corresponding increase in the concentration of II. Instead the degradation of I in alkaline solution is characterized by a complete loss of UV absorption spectra. This suggests that the pyrimidine ring is hydrolyzed. Figure 2 illustrates the probable reaction pathways for loss of I in alkaline solution proposed by Notari *et al.*[8] based on the work of Fox *et al.*[9]

Effect of light: At a concentration of 5 mg/ml in Elliots B and lactated Ringer's injection cytarabine exhibited no change in concentration over seven days, under fluorescent light, at room temperature and at 30°C. In 0.9% sodium chloride no decomposition occurred after 24 hours, but a 3% loss at room temperature, and a 6% loss at 30°C, was observed over seven days.[10] Benvenuto *et al.*[11] studied the stability of cytarabine (2 mg/ml) in glass and PVC bags (Viaflex, Baxter) in 5%

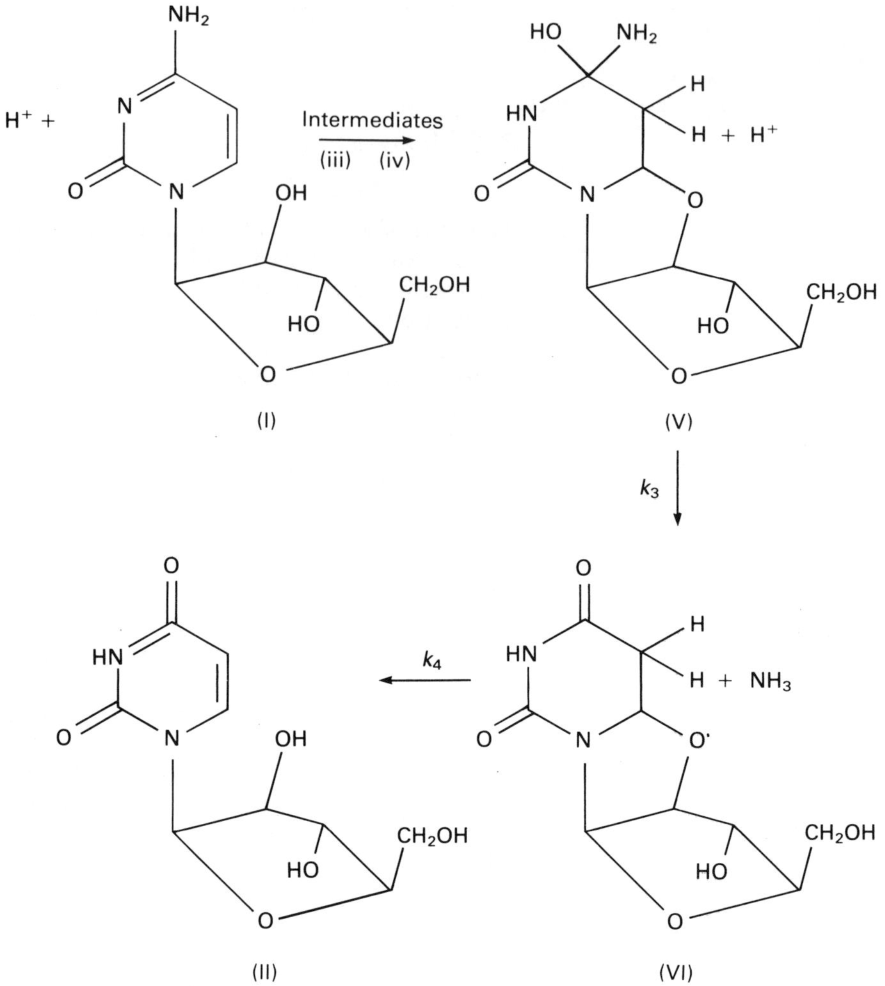

Figure 1: *Proposed mechanism for the acid catalysed degradation of cytarabine*[8]

glucose stored at room temperature and exposed to normal daylight. Results showed that cytarabine was stable ($< 10\%$ degradation) for 24 hours. These data indicate that photodegradation of cytarabine does not appear to be significant.

Effect of temperature: At a concentration of 800 mg/l, one group suggests that cytarabine in 0.9% sodium chloride and 5% glucose, showed no significant loss of activity over a period of 13 days,[4] whereas at a concentration of 500 mg/l, in the same solvents, another group indicated that cytarabine is stable for up to 48 hours.[5]

Gannon and Sesin[12] studied the stability of cytarabine in glass and polypropylene syringes at 25°C and 5°C. Results

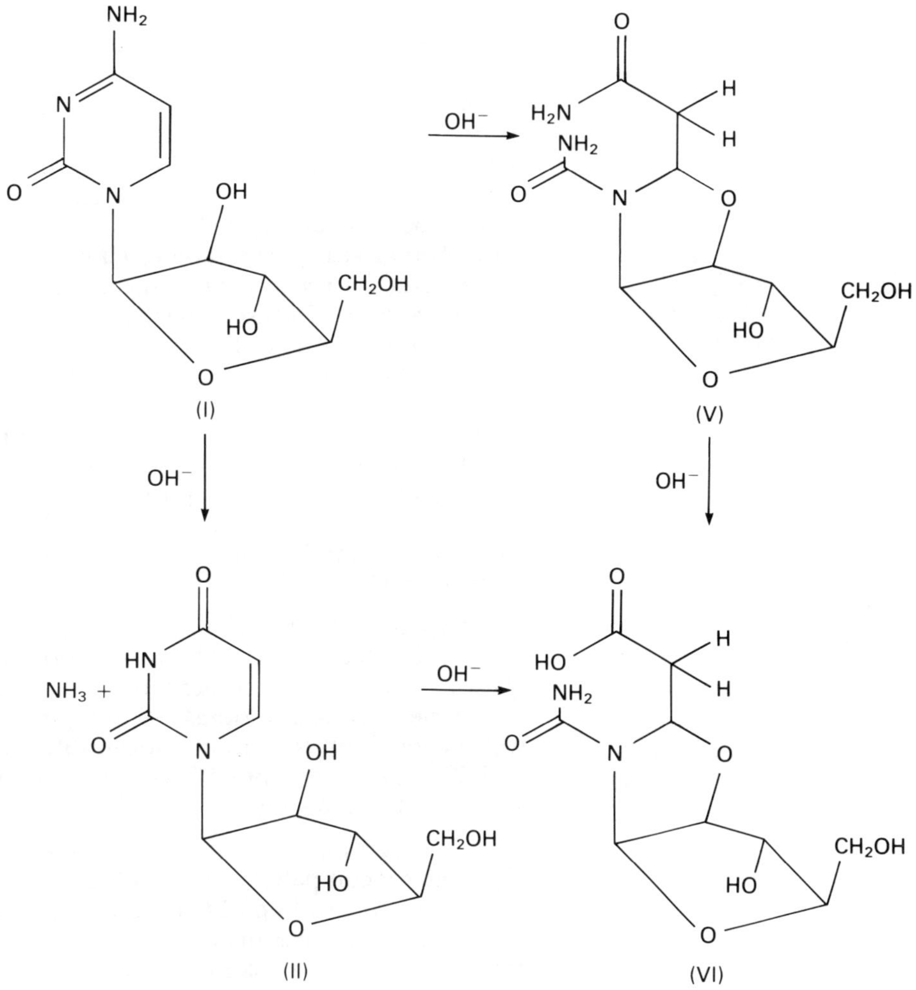

Figure 2: *Proposed mechanism for the degradation of cytarabine in alkaline solution*[8]

showed that cytarabine 20 mg/ml was more stable at 5°C in glass than plastic. The maximum decrease in potency over the seven day period of study in any of the containers was 2.9%. However, in that study, cytarabine concentration was measured using ultraviolet spectrophotometric assay. High-performance liquid chromatographic (HPLC) assay is a more accurate, specific and reliable method of determining drug concentration. Those authors indicated that further study was warranted using HPLC assay to confirm the overall stability of cytarabine.

Munson *et al.*[13] studied the stability of cytarabine in 5% glucose and glucose/saline in glass and PVC containers, with added sodium bicarbonate, at 22 and 8°C. Stability in water for injections in plastic syringes (Pharmaseal) was also studied at 22, 8 and −10°C. Results showed that in plastic syringes cytarabine, 20 mg/ml and 50 mg/ml, was chemically stable for one week at all temperatures studied. Addition of sodium bicarbonate, 50 mEq/L, to solutions had no effect on the chemical stability of cytarabine for at least one week at either at 22 or 8°C.[13] In a recently published study, Weir and Ireland[14] observed that cytarabine 100 mg in 5 ml, 500 mg in 10 ml and 1 g in 20 ml in polypropylene syringes was chemically stable for at least 30 days at 4 and 21°C.

In another study, cytarabine, 40 mg/ml and 80 mg/ml, reconstituted with water for injections, was shown to be stable in 5 ml Becton Dickinson plastic syringes for at least 15 days when stored at 4 and 25°C and for seven days at 37°C, however storage at −20°C resulted in precipitation.[5] Kirk *et al.*[15] noted that freezing cyclophosphamide in polypropylene syringes resulted in contraction of the plunger and seepage of the drugs past the barrel. Although this probably represents a negligible drug loss it is possible the potential risk of microbial contamination is unacceptable. For this reason freezing of cytarabine in polypropylene syringes is not recommended.

Container compatibility: Cytarabine is compatible with glass, PVC and polypropylene[12,13]. Adsorption of cytarabine on to glass has not been documented. Adsorption on to PVC is negligible at concentrations ≥0.5 mg/ml.[5] In clinical practice, when cytarabine is used at concentrations between 0.5 mg/ml and 20 mg/ml, adsorptive losses during storage and delivery are likely to be negligible.

Compatibility with other drugs: Cytarabine appears to be physically incompatible with methotrexate sodium,[4] 5-fluorouracil and heparin sodium.[16] Cytarabine is compatible with prednisolone sodium, sodium bicarbonate and vincristine sulphate.[16]

Stability in clinical practice

Cytarabine appears to be chemically stable for at least one week, and possibly one month, when reconstituted with water for injections, the enclosed diluent (with Cytosar), 5% glucose and/or sodium chloride when stored at 4°C.[5,13] It is important to note that bacterially contaminated intrathecal injections could pose very grave risks and consequently such solutions should be administered as soon as possible after reconstitution.[17]

4 Clinical Use

Main indications: Induction of clinical remission and/or maintenance therapy in patients with acute myeloid leukaemia, acute non-lymphoblastic leukaemias, acute lymphoblastic leukaemias, blast crises of chronic myeloid leukaemia and diffuse histiocytic lymphomas (non-Hodgkin's lymphomas of high malignancy).[6]

Dosage for Alexan: For remission induction the dose is 100 to 200 mg/m²/day or 3 to 6 mg/kg/day. For remission maintenance the following doses are recommended:

- ▼ Leukaemias: 75 to 100 mg/m²/day or 1.5–3 mg/kg/day for five consecutive days once a month or for one day each week.
- ▼ CNS leukaemias: 10 to 30 mg/m² three times weekly, intrathecally.

Dosage for Alexan 100: Evidence suggests that the maximum tolerated dose is 3 g/m² every 12 hours for six days. High dose Alexan is reserved for the treatment of resistant or refractory cases of leukaemia.[1]

Dosage for Cytosar: For continuous treatment a dose of 2 mg/kg/day for 10 days, as a starting dose is given by bolus injection. If no antileukaemic effect and no toxicity is observed the dose may be increased to 4 mg/kg/day until a therapeutic response or toxicity occurs. Alternatively, 0.5 to 1.0 mg/kg/day may be given as an infusion of up to 24 hours duration. After 10 days the dose may be increased to 2 mg/kg/day subject to toxicity. Treatment is continued until remission or toxicity occurs.[2]

For intermittent treatment an intravenous dosage of 3 to 5 mg/kg/day is administered on each of five consecutive days. After a two to nine day rest period a further course is given. Treatment is continued until a response or toxicity occurs.[2] Remissions which have been induced by cytarabine may be maintained by intravenous or subcutaneous injection of 1 mg/kg once or twice weekly.

5 Preparation of Injection

Reconstitution: The contents of the vial (Cytosar) may be reconstituted with water for injections, 0.9% sodium chloride or 5% glucose. When reconstituted with the accompanying diluent (water for injections containing 0.9% benzyl alcohol as preservative) addition of the diluent and gentle shaking of the contents will produce a solution containing 20 mg/ml (100 mg vial) or 50 mg/ml (500 mg vial) of cytarabine.[2]

Bolus administration: Alexan is administered by intravenous, intrathecal, intramuscular and subcutaneous injection. For intrathecal injection it is recommended that 5 to 8 ml of cerebrospinal fluid (CSF) is drawn up, mixed with the injection solution in the syringe and slowly re-injected. Intramuscular and subcutaneous injections are usually used only in maintenance therapy.[1]

Subcutaneous injection of Alexan 100 is not recommended at present due to a lack of clinical data. Intrathecal or intramuscular use of Alexan 100 is contraindicated due to slight hypertonicity of the formulation.[1] Cytarabine (Cytosar) may be administered by intravenous infusion or injection or by subcutaneous injection.[2]

Infusion: To prepare an infusion Alexan can be added to 0.9% sodium chloride or 5% glucose solution. In high dose schedules Alexan 100 should be administered by continuous intravenous infusion in either 0.9% sodium chloride or 5% glucose solution. To reduce toxicity the duration of the infusion should not be less than one hour.[1] Continuous infusions of cytarabine have ranged from eight to 12 hours to 120 to 168 hours.[1,18] Kreis *et al.*[19] investigated a low dose infusion given over 21 days. Slevin *et al.*[20] compared intravenous and subcutaneous infusions. Results in that study showed that subcutaneous infusion was well tolerated without any local discomfort or excoriation.[20] Continuous infusions (compared to bolus doses) show more pronounced gastrointestinal side-effects.[1]

Gloves for handling: Rubber gloves are recommended.

Extravasation: Cytarabine is mildly irritant and is not known to cause any serious tissue injury when extravasated. If necessary the standard extravasation procedures may be followed.

6 Destruction of Drugs or Contaminated Articles

Incineration: 1000°C.[3,4,5]

Chemical: Hydrochloric acid/24 hours.[3,4,5]

Contact with skin: Wash with water, or soap and water. If the eyes are contaminated immediate irrigation with sodium chloride 0.9% should be carried out.[3,4,5]

References

1. ABPI Data Sheet Compendium 1989/1990. (1989). Datapharm Publications Ltd, London, pp. 1217–1219.
2. ABPI Data Sheet Compendium 1989/1990. (1989). Datapharm Publications Ltd, London, pp. 1656–1657.
3. Personal communication, David Bull Laboratories. Unpublished Data.
4. Personal communication, Pfizer Ltd. Unpublished data.
5. Personal communication, Upjohn Ltd. Unpublished data.
6. Anon. (1989). *The extra pharmacopeoia*, 29th edn, Reynolds J.E.F. (ed.), The Pharmaceutical Press, London, pp. 619–621.
7. Notari, R.E. (1967). A mechanism for the hydrolytic deamination of cytosine arabinoside in aqueous buffer. *J. Pharm. Sci.* **56**, 804–809.
8. Notari, R.E. *et al.* (1972). Arabinosylcytosine stability in aqueous solutions: pH profile and shelf-life predictions. *J. Pharm. Sci.* **61**, 1189–1196.
9. Fox, J.J. *et al.* (1966). Nucleosides XXXVI. Transformation of arabinopyrimidine nucleosides (1). *Tetrahedron Lett.* **40**, 4927–4934.
10. Cradock, J.C. *et al.* (1978) Evaluation of some pharmaceutical aspects of intrathecal methotrexate sodium, cytarabine and hydrocortisone sodium succinate. *Am. J. Hosp. Pharm.* **35**, 402–406.

11. Benvenuto, J.A. *et al.* (1981). Stability and compatibility of antitumour agents in glass and plastic containers. *Am. J. Hosp. Pharm.* **38**, 1914–1918.
12. Gannon, P.M. and Sesin, G.P. (1983). Stability of cytarabine following repackaging in plastic syringes and glass containers. *Am. J. Intravenous Ther. Clin. Nutrition* **10**, 11–16.
13. Munson, J.W. *et al.* (1982). Cytosine arabinoside stability in intravenous admixtures with sodium bicarbonate and in plastic syringes. *Drug Intell. Clin. Pharm.* **16**, 765–767.
14. Weir, P.J. and Ireland, D.S. (1990). Chemical stability of cytarabine and vinblastine injection. *Br. J. Pharm. Pract.* **12**, 53–56.
15. Kirk, B. *et al.* (1984). Chemical stability of cyclophosphamide injection: The effect of low temperature storage and microwave thawing. *Br. J. Parent. Ther.* 90–97.
16. Trissel, L.A. (1988). *Handbook of injectable drugs*, 5th edn, American Society of Hospital Pharmacists, Bethesda, Maryland, USA.
17. Sarubbi, F.A. *et al.* (1978). Nosocomial meningitis and bacteraemia due to contaminated Amphotericin B. *J. Am. Med. Assoc.* **35**, 402–406.
18. Spriggs, D.R. *et al.* (1985). Continuous infusion of high dose cytarabine a phase I and pharmacological study. *Cancer Res.* **45**, 3932–3936.
19. Kreis, W. *et al.* (1985). Pharmacokinetics of low dose 1-β-D arabinofuranosylcytosine given by continuous IV infusion over 21 days. *Cancer Res.* **45**, 6498–6501.
20. Slevin, M.L. *et al.* (1983). Subcutaneous infusion of cytosine arabinoside – A practical alternative to intravenous infusion. *Cancer Chemother. Pharmacol.* **10**, 112–114.

Prepared by M.J. Wood.

DACARBAZINE

1 General Details

Approved name: Dacarbazine.

Proprietary name: DTIC-Dome.

Manufacturer or supplier: Bayer (UK) Ltd.

Presentation and formulation details: A colourless or ivory-coloured powder in amber glass vials containing 100 mg or 200 mg dacarbazine as the citrate salt. The 100 mg vial contains 100 mg citric acid and 50 mg mannitol. The 200 mg vial contains 100 mg citric acid and 37.5 mg mannitol. The vials do not contain any preservatives.

Storage and shelf-life of unopened container: Three years stored at 2 to 8°C and protected from light.

2 Chemistry

Type: Triazene, alkylating agent.

Molecular structure: 5-(3,3-dimethyl-1-1-triazeno) imidazole-4-carboxamide.

$$\text{HN} \quad \text{N} \quad \text{CONH}_2 \quad \text{N}=\text{N}-\text{N(CH}_3)_2$$

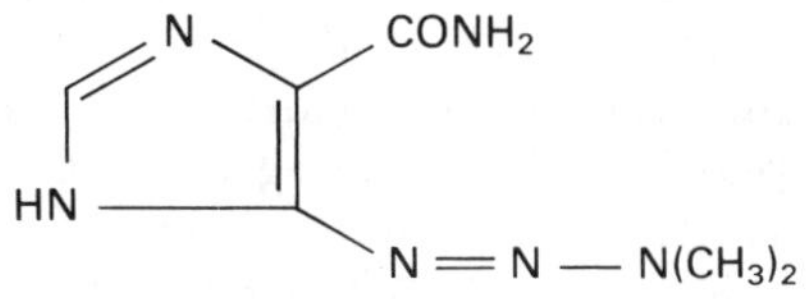

Molecular weight: 182.2.

Solubility: 1 mg/ml in water and 60 mg/ml in 10% citric acid.

3. Stability Profile

Physical and chemical stability

Dacarbazine is relatively stable after reconstitution and further dilution, the reconstituted drug being stable for at least 72 hours if stored at 2 to 8°C.[1] After further dilution in 0.9% sodium chloride or 5% glucose, there is less than 1% degradation after 24 hours storage at 4°C, if protected from light.[1,2]

Dacarbazine is very sensitive to daylight.[3-6] Exposure to sunlight causes rapid degradation.[4] However, exposure to artificial (fluorescent) light or diffuse daylight is far less detrimental. Kirk,[4] in a detailed study, has shown that approximately 4 to 6% losses were recorded during administration under conditions of 'normal' room lighting (diffuse daylight and fluorescent light), whilst solutions exposed to strong daylight showed losses of the order of 12% in 90 minutes. Photodegradation is indicated by a colour change from yellow to pink.

Degradation pathways: The mechanisms described by Kirk[4] have been elucidated by Horton and Stevens.[7] The degradation route of dacarbazine (DTIC) in solutions of different pH either exposed to daylight or maintained in the dark are shown in Figure 1; the principal degradation products are 5-diazoimidazole-4-carboxamide (DIAZO-IC:II), 2-azahypoxanthine (III), a metastable intermediate carbene moeity (IV) and 4-carbamoylimidazolium-5-olate (V).

The primary degradation product of photolysis is 5-diazoimidazole-4-carboxamide (DIAZO-IC). Further degradation then occurs to conjugated polymers, which give rise to the pink coloration. It has been suggested that these polymers are responsible for localized side-effects at the site of injection.[3] This has not been confirmed.

Container compatibility: Dacarbazine is compatible with PVC containers and administration sets[4,5,8] and with Amberset (Avon Medical Ltd).[4] There is no further information on

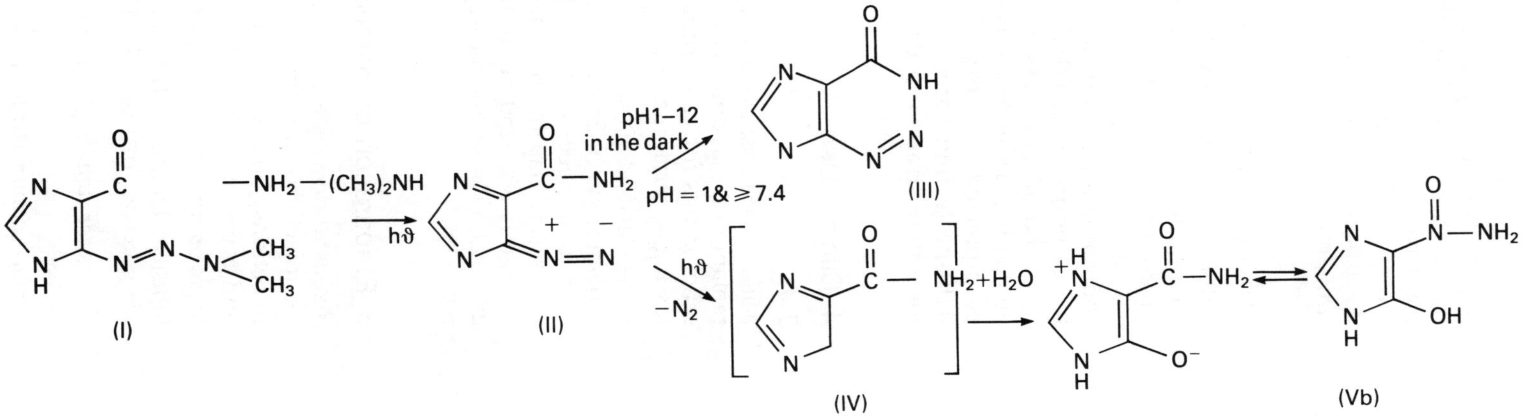

Figure 1: *The degradation route of dacarbazine (DTIC) in solutions of different pH either exposed to daylight or maintained in the dark*

dacarbazine's compatibility with other delivery systems such as plastic syringes.[5]

Compatibility with other drugs: Dacarbazine forms an immediate precipitate with hydrocortisone sodium succinate, but not with hydrocortisone sodium phosphate nor with lignocaine 1 to 2%.[9] Dacarbazine is compatible with heparin in 5% dextrose.[9] A white precipitate has been observed when tubing containing dacarbazine (25 mg/ml) was flushed with heparin (100 units/ml).[10]

Stability in clinical practice

After reconstitution with water for injections, the resulting 10 mg/ml solution is stable in the vial for 72 hours at 4°C, protected from light, or eight hours at normal temperature.[1,2,5]

   This solution can be further diluted in 5% glucose or 0.9% sodium chloride infusions and the resulting solution is stable for 24 hours at 2 to 8°C. Dacarbazine is very sensitive to UV light and all unnecessary exposure to daylight should be avoided. During administration, the infusion container should be protected from exposure to daylight. The use of a UV light-protecting administration set should be recommended for administration in daylight conditions.[4]

4 Clinical Use

Type of cytotoxic: Alkylating agent.

Main indications: As a single agent in metastatic malignant melanoma, sarcoma, Hodgkin's disease. In combination with other drugs for carcinoma of colon, ovary, breast, lung, testicular teratoma and some solid tumours in children.

Dosage and administration: 2 to 4.5 mg/kg/day for 10 days repeated every 28 days. 650 to 1450 mg/m^2 repeated every four to six weeks. 750 to 1200 mg/m^2 repeated every 21 days. 250 mg/m^2/day for five days repeated every 21 days. Paediatric dosage is 200–250 mg/m^2/day for 5 days, repeated every 28 days. (These are the regimens used at The Royal Marsden Hospital.)

5 Preparation of Injection

Reconstitution: The 100 mg vial is reconstituted with 9.9 ml water for injections and the 200 mg vial with 19.7 ml water for injections, both giving a final concentration of 10 mg/ml and a pH of 3.0 to 4.0.

Bolus administration: Inject slowly over 1 to 2 minutes.

Infusion: Dilute in 125 to 250 ml 0.9% sodium chloride or 5% glucose. Infuse over 15 to 30 minutes.

Gloves for handling: Rubber, polyethylene or thick PVC should be used.

Extravasation: Moderately damaging. No specific antidote.

6 Destruction of Drug or Contaminated Articles

Incineration: 500°C.

Chemical: The solution can be digested in 10% sulphuric acid for 24 hours, then washed down the sink with copious amounts of water.

Contact with skin: Wash with water.

References

1. ABPI Data Sheet Compendium 1989/90. (1989). Datapharm Publications Ltd, London, pp. 125–126.
2. Trissell, L.S. (1988). *Handbook of injectable drugs*, 5th edn, American Society of Hospital Pharmacists, Bethesda, Maryland, USA.
3. Baird, S.M. and Willoughby, M.L.N. (1978). Photo-degradation of dacarbazine. *Lancet,* **ii**, 681.
4. Kirk, B. (1987). The evaluation of a light-protecting giving set. *Intensive Ther. & Clin. Monitor.* **8**, 78–86.
5. Personal communication, Bayer (UK) Ltd. Unpublished data.
6. Personal communication. (1988). Institute of Cancer Research, London. Unpublished data.
7. Horton, J.K. and Stevens, M.F.G. (1981). A new light on the photodecomposition of the antitumour drug DTIC. *J. Pharm. Pharmacol.* **33**, 808–811.
8. Benvenuto, J.A. *et al.* (1981). Stability and compatibility of antitumour agents in glass and plastic containers. *Am. J. Hosp. Pharm.* **38**, 1914–1918.
9. Dorr, R.T. (1979). Incompatibilities with parenteral anticancer drugs. *Am. J. Intravenous Ther.* **6**, 42–52.
10. Nelson, R.W. *et al.* (1987). Visual incompatibility of dacarbazine and heparin. *Am. J. Hosp. Pharm.* **44**, 2028.

Prepared by T. Root and K. Patel.

DACTINOMYCIN

1 General Details

Approved names: Dactinomycin, actinomycin D.

Proprietary name: Cosmegen Lyovac.

Manufacturer or supplier: Merck, Sharpe & Dohme Ltd.

Presentation and formulation details: Yellow lyophilized powder in vial, containing 500 µg dactinomycin. Each vial contains 20 mg mannitol.

Storage and shelf-life of unopened container: Five years when stored in cool, dry place protected from light.

2 Chemistry

Type: Antibiotic.

Molecular structure: Actinomycin(thr-val-pro-sar-meval).

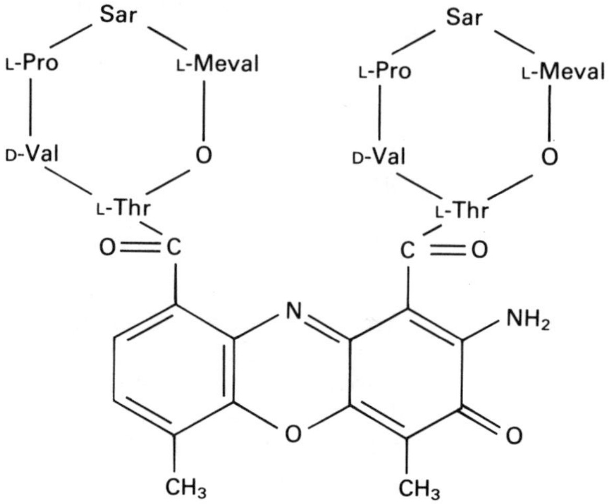

$$
\begin{array}{cc}
\text{Sar} & \text{Sar} \\
\text{L-Pro} \quad \text{L-Meval} & \text{L-Pro} \quad \text{L-Meval} \\
\text{D-Val} \quad \text{O} & \text{D-Val} \quad \text{O} \\
\text{L-Thr} & \text{L-Thr} \\
O{=}C & C{=}O \\
\end{array}
$$

Molecular weight: 1255.5.

Solubility: Soluble in water.

3 Stability Profile

Physical and chemical stability

Degradation in aqueous solution is pH dependent. The pH of reconstituted drug is 5.5 to 7.0 and it is most stable between pH 5 and 7. One report indicates approximately 2 to 3% degradation in 6 days at 25°C at these pH values (30 µg/ml).[1] At pH 9.0, 80% loss was noted under the same conditions.[1]

Degradation pathways: Alkaline conditions – ring opening of the acridine-like centre.[2]

Physical: Degradation is reduced at lower temperatures. In aqueous solution, degradation at 2 to 6°C is negligible over a 6 day period.[1]

Container compatibility: Syringes – no information available. Dactinomycin is reported to be compatible with glass and PVC containers for infusions.[3]

No information is available on the compatibility of administration sets, but it should be noted that dactinomycin is compatible with PVC.[2]

There is evidence of dactinomycin binding to certain types of in-line filters.[4] For example, when 500 µg was diluted in 500 ml infusion fluid a total of 67 µg (approximately 13%) was subsequently bound to the in-line cellulose acetate membrane filter. Binding to polycarbonate filters has also been reported.[4]

Compatibility with other drugs and excipients: Incompatible with benzyl alcohol and other preservatives; avoid preserved diluents for reconstitution.

Stability in clinical practice
The drug is relatively stable after reconstitution in water for injections and may be stored at 2 to 6°C for seven days. The drug is also reasonably stable after further dilution in 0.9% sodium chloride or 5% glucose showing less than 10% degradation after 24 hours at ambient temperature.[3] It should be protected from daylight during storage. The reconstituted drug is also stable when frozen.[5]

4 Clinical Use

Type of cytotoxic: Cytotoxic antibiotic.

Main indications: Wilms tumour; rhabdomyosarcoma; carcinoma of testis or uterus.

Dosage: 15 µg/kg for up to five days.

5 Preparation of Injection

Reconstitution: Add 1.1 ml water for injections and shake to dissolve. The injection may be stored for up to seven days at 2 to 6°C.

Bolus administration: Inject into the tubing of a fast-running infusion of saline or glucose.

Infusion: Add to up to 500 ml 0.9% sodium chloride or 5% glucose. The infusion may be stored for 24 hours at 2 to 6°C.

Stability in plastic syringes: No information available.

Gloves for handling: Rubber gloves should be used.

Extravasation: Very damaging; no antidote known.

6 Destruction of Drug or Contaminated Articles

Incineration: 800°C.

Chemical: 10% trisodium phosphate in excess, or 20% sodium hydroxide.

Contact with skin: Wash in water or sodium phosphate solution.

References

1. Crevar, G.E. and Slotnick, I.J. (1964). A note on the stability of actinomycin D. *J. Pharm. Pharmacol.* **16**, 429.
2. Johnson, A.W. (1960). The chemistry of antinomycin D and related compounds. *Annal. New York Acad. Sci.* **89**, 336–341.
3. Benvenuto, J.A. *et al.* (1981). Stability and compatibility of antitumour agents in glass and plastic containers. *Am. J. Hosp. Pharm.*, **38**, 1914–1918.
4. Rusmin, S. *et al.* (1977). Effect of inline filtration on the potency of drugs administered intravenously. *Am. J. Hosp. Pharm.* **34**, 1071–1074.
5. Bosanquet, A.G. (1986). Stability of solutions of antineoplastic agents during preparation and storage for *in vitro* assays II. Assay methods, adriamycin and other antitumour antibiotics. *Cancer Chemother. Pharmacol.* **17**, 1–10.

Prepared by M.C. Allwood

DAUNORUBICIN

1 General Details

Approved name: Daunorubicin.

Proprietary name: Cerubicin.

Manufacturer or supplier: Rhône-Poulenc UK Ltd.

Presentation and formulation details: Sterile, pyrogen-free, orange-red, freeze-dried powder in vials of 20 mg of daunorubicin hydrochloride, with mannitol. There are no preservatives in the preparation.[1]

Storage and shelf-life of unopened container: Dry, unopened vials expire three years from the date of manufacture when stored in a dry place protected from sunlight. Vials of daunorubicin are stored at room temperature.

2 Chemistry

Type: Daunorubicin is a cytotoxic antibiotic consisting of an aminosugar moiety linked through a glycosidic bond to the C7 of a tetracyclic aglycone, daunosamine. It forms a stable complex with DNA and interferes with the synthesis of nucleic acids. The cytotoxic effects of daunorubicin are most marked on cells in the S phase.[2]

Molecular structure:

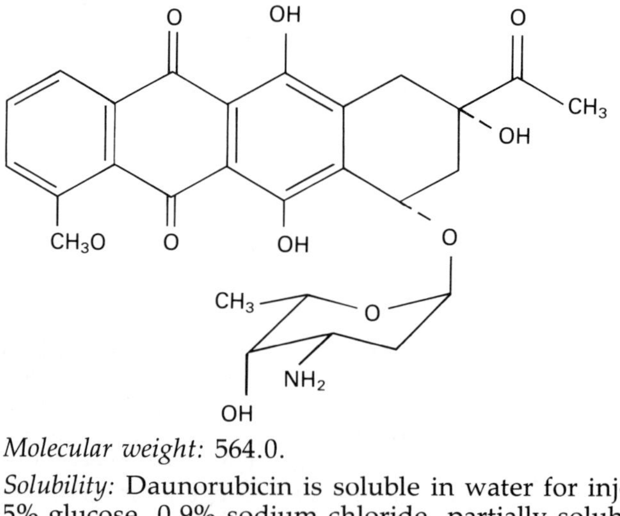

Molecular weight: 564.0.

Solubility: Daunorubicin is soluble in water for injections, 5% glucose, 0.9% sodium chloride, partially soluble in methanol and ethanol and practically insoluble in chloroform, ether and organic solvents.[2]

3 Stability Profile

Physical and chemical stability

The manufacturer states that the reconstituted solution is stable for up to 24 hours, at 2 to 8°C, when protected from bright light. The literature reveals that daunorubicin may be chemically stable for longer periods although few data have been published.[3–5]

The stability of daunorubicin depends on a number of factors. Degradation in aqueous solution is pH-dependent. Daunorubicin is also light sensitive and adsorbs on to glass and certain plastics.

Effect of pH: Daunorubicin becomes progressively more stable as the pH of the drug fluid admixture becomes more acidic (pH 7.4 to 4.5).[4] Maximum stability is observed at about pH 5.[6]

Decomposition in acidic solution has been studied by Beijnen *et al.*[7] Acidic hydrolysis of daunorubicin (pH less than 3.5), shown in Figure 1, yields a red-coloured, water-insoluble aglycone, daunorubicinone and a water-soluble amino sugar, daunosamine. The rate of cleavage of the glycosidic bond in acidic media is strongly dependent on structural modifications in the amino sugar moiety and unaffected by structural modifications in the aglycone portion of the molecule. As doxorubicin and daunorubicin both possess daunosamine as the amino sugar moiety, the rate of degradation of these two analogues is similar in acidic solution.[7]

At pH values above 3.5, two major degradation products are formed, both of which are aglycones, 7,8-dehydro-9,10-desacetyl-daunorubicinone and 7,8–9,10-bisanhydrodauno-rubicinone.[6,8] The proposed mechanism for this degradation is shown in Figure 2.

On addition to strongly alkaline solution a colour change from red to a deep blue-purple is observed and rapid degradation of daunorubicin occurs. Analysis of the decomposition of daunorubicin at pH 8.0 showed formation of seven possible degradation products, the three major degradation products being, 7,8–9,10-bisanhydrodaunorubi-cinone (I), 7 deoxydaunorubicinone (II) and 7,8,-dehydro-9,10-desacetyldaunorubicinone III. The structures of these products are shown in Figure 3. Low yields of the remaining four compounds prevented full characterization and structure elucidation.[5–9]

The rate of degradation of the anthracyclines in alkaline media is affected by structural differences in the aglycone portion of the molecule and unaffected by structural differences in the amino sugar moiety.[8] Daunorubicin has been observed to be more stable than doxorubicin in alkaline solution.[8] As the only difference between doxorubicin and daunorubicin is a C14 proton in daunorubicin versus a hydroxyl group in doxorubicin this structural difference must hold the key to the differences in stability of these two drugs.[8]

Effect of light: Data on the kinetics of degradation of doxorubicin in fluorescent light have been published[10] but, until recently, there were no data available for daunorubicin. Results from a study in which the rates of photodegradation of doxorubicin, daunorubicin and epirubicin were compared indicated that the rate of photodegradation of all three analogues was similar.[11] This suggests that the rate of photodegradation of daunorubicin

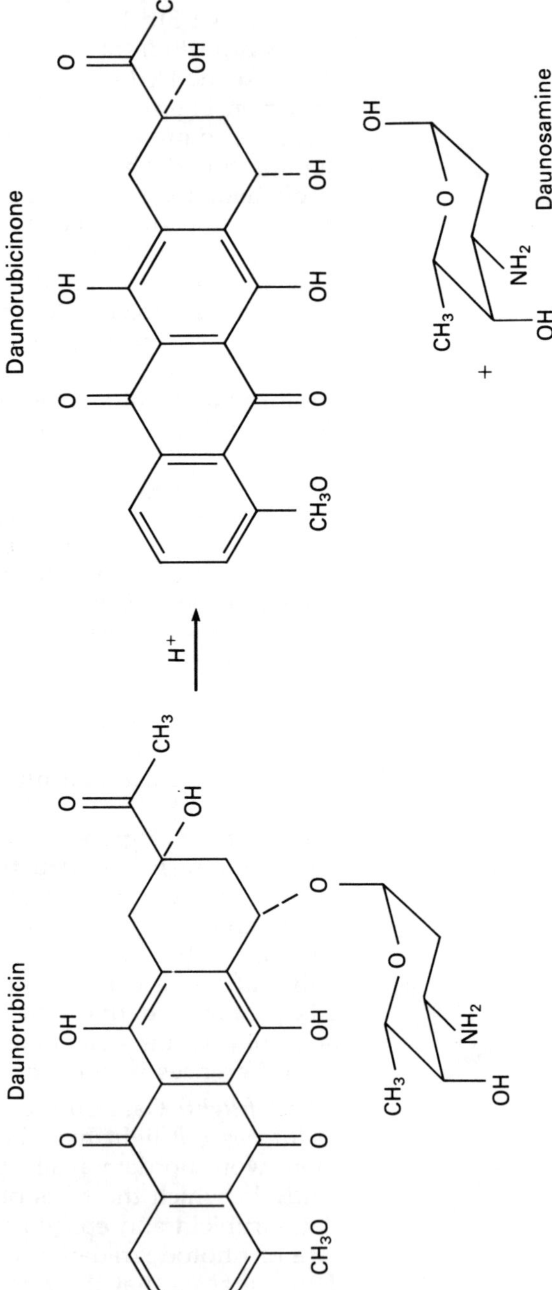

Figure 1: *Degradation pathway of daunorubicin in acidic solution*

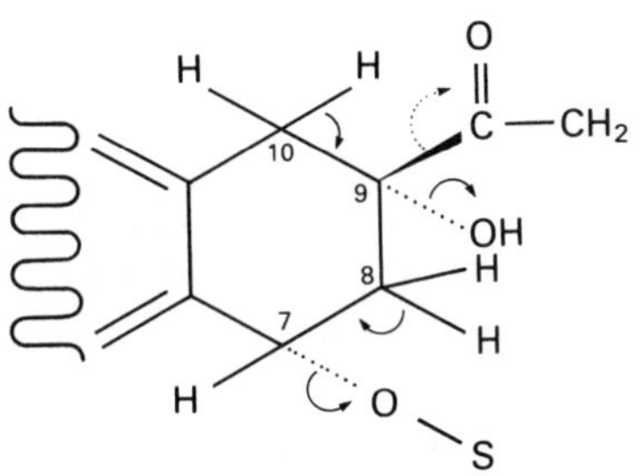

Figure 2: *Degradation scheme of daunorubicin (pH ca4). S refers to the daunosamine sugar moiety*[6]

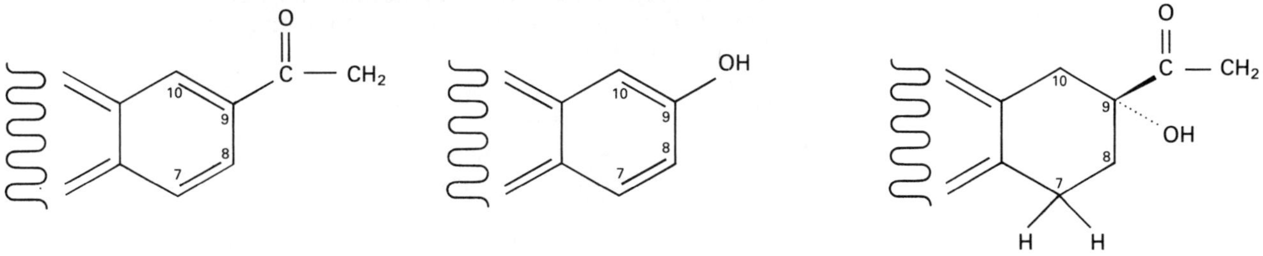

(I)　　　　　　　　　　　(II)　　　　　　　　　　　(III)

Figure 3: *Structure of the major degradation products of daunorubicin at pH 8.0*[9]

may be significant at concentrations below 100 µg/ml if solutions are exposed to light for sufficient time. However, at higher concentrations, such as those used for cancer chemotherapy (≥ 500 µg/ml), no special precautions are necessary to protect freshly prepared solutions of daunorubicin from light.[11]

Effect of temperature: Studies designed to investigate the effect of temperature on the rate of degradation of daunorubicin in buffers at pH 8.0 and pH 1.5 between 40 and 60°C showed that the Arrhenius equation was obeyed.[6] Results from stability studies at room temperature (normally 25°C), in the refrigerator (about 4°C) or in the freezer (about −20°C) are presented below.

Poochikian *et al.*[4] observed that daunorubicin (20 µg/ml) was stable for 72 hours in 5% glucose and 0.9% sodium chloride in glass containers at 21°C. In that study, solutions were not protected from light and, at the low concentrations used, photodegradation may represent a considerable proportion of the overall degradation observed. Conversely, in a well-controlled study, where the solutions were protected from light, daunorubicin was stable in polypropylene tubes, for 28 days in 5% glucose (pH 4.7), 3.3% glucose with 0.3% sodium chloride (pH 4.4) and 0.9% sodium chloride (pH 7.0) at 25°C.[5] Daunorubicin has also been reported to be stable for seven days at room temperature.[3] In another study, daunorubicin was reported to be stable (loss in potency of less than 10%) in 5% glucose (pH 4.36) and 0.9% sodium chloride (pH 5.20 and 6.47) in PVC minibags for at least 43 days at 25, 4 and −20°C.[12] Repeated freezing and thawing of solutions stored at −20°C did not cause degradation. In the same study, daunorubicin was also reported to be stable for at least 43 days when reconstituted with water for injections and stored in polypropylene syringes at 4°C.[12]

Container compatibility: Daunorubicin is compatible with polypropylene, PVC and glass.[12] Daunorubicin adsorbs on to glass but not on to siliconized glass or polypropylene.[13] In clinical practice, when daunorubicin is used at concentrations of at least 500 µg/ml, adsorptive losses during storage and delivery are negligible.[12]

Compatibility with other drugs: Daunorubicin is incompatible with dexamethasone sodium phosphate and heparin sodium but is compatible with hydrocortisone sodium succinate.[1] The manufacturer recommends that no other drugs are mixed with daunorubicin.

Stability in clinical practice

Daunorubicin is compatible with polypropylene, PVC and glass.[12] Daunorubicin appears to be chemically stable for at least 28 days in PVC minibags containing 5% glucose and 0.9% sodium chloride stored at 4 and $-20°C$ and for at least 28 days in polypropylene syringes at 4°C.[12]

4 Clinical Use

Main indications: The treatment of acute leukaemia. In acute myeloblastic leukaemia, daunorubicin is used alone, or in combination with other cytotoxic drugs, at all stages of disease development. In acute lymphoblastic leukaemia, daunorubicin is a very active remission-inducing agent, but because of its toxicity and the availability of other treatments, its use is chiefly indicated in those cases which have proved resistant to treatment with other drugs. Its use in disseminated solid tumours has also aroused interest and its effectiveness has been demonstrated in some cases of disseminated neuroblastoma and rhabdomyosarcoma.[1]

Dosage and administration: The dosage of each individual injection may vary from 0.5 to 3 mg/kg. Doses of 0.5 to 1.0 mg/kg may be repeated at intervals of one or more days; doses of 2 mg/kg should be spaced four or more days apart; high doses of 2.5 or 3 mg/kg should only be given at seven to 14 day intervals. In acute myeloblastic leukaemia, each dose should be about 2 mg/kg, repeated at four to seven day intervals, according to the response. In acute lymphoblastic leukaemia, doses of 1 mg/kg may be repeated, according to tolerance and effect, at one to four day intervals.

For dosages calculated in terms of body surface area the manufacturer recommends a dose of 50 mg/m² (for adults) on alternate days, for a course of up to three injections. The number of injections required varies from patient to patient and must be determined in each case by response and tolerance. A dosage reduction of up to 50% is recommended in the elderly. The dosage for children over one year is the same as for adults and for children below one year, 75% of the adult dose is recommended.[14]

When administered with other cytotoxic agents with overlapping toxicity, dosage should be suitably reduced. A cumulative dose of 500 to 600 mg/m² should not be exceeded as the risk of irreversible congestive cardiac failure increases greatly.[1]

5 Preparation of Injection

Reconstitution: The contents of the 20 mg vial are reconstituted with 4 ml of water for injections. After addition of the diluent and gentle shaking, the contents of the vial will dissolve to produce a solution of 5 mg/ml.[1]

Bolus administration: Administration is by the intravenous route only. The manufacturers recommend that the calculated dose is further diluted with normal saline to give a final concentration of 1 mg/ml. This solution should be injected, over a 20 minute period, into the side arm of a freely-running intravenous infusion of 0.9% sodium chloride. This technique minimizes the risk of thrombosis or perivenous extravasation, which can lead to severe cellulitis or vesication.[1]

Infusion: Although daunorubicin has been used as a continuous infusion in a phase I trial in previously treated patients with leukaemia, no phase II evaluation was conducted because of somewhat limited antileukaemic activity in patients who had previously received other anthracycline therapy.[15]

Gloves for handling: Rubber gloves are recommended.

Extravasation: Daunorubicin is a potent vesicant. Facial flushing or erythematous streaking along the vein indicates the injection was too rapid. Should extravasation occur, the infusion should be stopped immediately and resumed in another vein. Appropriate treatment for the extravasated area should be commenced immediately.[1]

6 Destruction of Drug or Contaminated Articles

Incineration: 700°C.[14]

Chemical: Diluted sodium hypochlorite (1% available chlorine)/ 24 hours.[1]

Contact with skin: Wash with water, soap and water, or sodium bicarbonate solution. If the eyes are contaminated immediate irrigation with 0.9% sodium chloride should be carried out.[1]

References

1. Daunorubicin: Package Insert. (1989). Rhône-Poulenc UK Ltd, Rainham Road South, Dagenham, Essex, UK.
2. Anon. (1989). *The Extra Pharmacopoeia*, 29th edn, Reynolds J.E.F. (ed.), Pharmaceutical Press, London, p. 622.
3. Trissel, L.A. (1988). *Handbook of injectable drugs*, 5th edn, American Society of Hospital Pharmacists, Bethesda, Maryland, USA.
4. Poochikian, G.K. *et al.* (1981). Stability of anthracycline antitumour agents in four infusion fluids. *Am. J. Hosp. Pharm.* **38**, 483–486.

5. Beijnen, J.H. *et al.* (1985a). Stability of anthracycline antitumour agents in infusion fluids. *J. Parent. Sci. Technol.* **39**, 220–222.
6. Beijnen, J.H. *et al.* (1986a). Aspects of the degradation kinetics of daunorubicin in aqueous solution. *Int. J. Pharm.* **31**, 75–82.
7. Beijnen, J.H. *et al.* (1985b). Aspects of the chemical stability of daunorubicin and seven other anthracyclines in acidic solution. *Pharm. Weekbl. (Sci. Edn)* **7**, 109–116.
8. Beijnen, J.H. *et al.* (1986b). Aspects of the degradation kinetics of doxorubicin in aqueous solution. *Int. J. Pharm.* **32**, 123–131.
9. Beijnen, J.H. *et al.* (1987). Structure elucidation and characterization of daunorubicin degradation products. *Int. J. Pharm.* **34**, 247–257.
10. Tavoloni, N. *et al.* (1980). Photolytic degradation of adriamycin. Communications: *J. Pharm. Pharmacol.* **32**, 860–862.
11. Wood, M.J. *et al.* (1990). Photodegradation of doxorubicin, daunorubicin and epirubicin measured by high-performance liquid chromatography. *J. Clin. Pharm. Ther.* (In Press).
12. Wood, M.J. *et al.* (1990). Stability of doxorubicin, daunorubicin and epirubicin in plastic syringes and minibags. *J. Clin. Pharm. Ther.* (In Press).
13. Bosanquet, A.G. (1986). Stability of solutions of antineoplastic agents during preparation and storage for *in vitro* assays. II. Assay methods, adriamycin and the other antitumour antibiotics. *Cancer Chemother. Pharmacol.* **17**, 1–10.
14. Personal communication, Rhône Polenc UK Ltd. Unpublished data.
15. Legha, S.S. *et al.* (1987). Anthracyclines: In Cancer chemotherapy by infusion. Lokich J.J. (ed.), MTP Press Ltd, Lancaster.

Prepared by M.J. Wood

DOXORUBICIN

1 General Details

Approved name: Doxorubicin.

Proprietary name: Adriamycin (Doxorubicin Rapid Dissolution).

Manufacturer or supplier: Farmitalia Carlo Erba Ltd.

Presentation and formulation details: Doxorubicin Rapid Dissolution: Sterile, pyrogen-free, orange-red, freeze-dried powder in vials containing 10 mg, 20 mg and 50 mg of doxorubicin hydrochloride with lactose and hydroxybenzoate. The inclusion of methylhydroxybenzoate 0.02% (which is a sub-preservative concentration) is to prevent gel formation, which used to occur occasionally on reconstitution of Adriamycin. Adriamycin has been replaced by Doxorubicin Rapid Dissolution.[1]

Doxorubicin solution for injection sterile, red, mobile solution in vials of 10 and 50 mg, each containing doxorubicin hydrochloride as a 2 mg/ml solution in 0.9% sodium chloride injection. The solution is adjusted to pH 3 with 0.5 M hydrochloric acid.[2]

Storage and shelf-life of unopened container: Doxorubicin rapid Dissolution: Dry, unopened vials expire three years from the date of manufacture when stored in a dry place protected from light.

Doxorubicin solution for injection should be stored in the refrigerator (2 to 8°C). Vials expire 18 months from the date of manufacture when stored at this temperature. Once removed from the refrigerator, the shelf-life is one month.[3]

2 Chemistry

Type: A cytotoxic antibiotic consisting of an aminosugar, daunosamine, linked through a glycosidic bond to the C7 of a tetracyclic aglycone, doxorubicinone. Doxorubicin may act by forming a stable complex with DNA and interfering with the synthesis of nucleic acids. It is most active against cells in the S phase.[4]

Molecular structure:

Molecular weight: 580.0.

Solubility: Doxorubicin is soluble in water for injections, 5% glucose and 0.9% sodium chloride, partially soluble in methanol and ethanol and practically insoluble in chloroform, ether and other organic solvents.[4]

3 Stability Profile

Physical and chemical stability: The manufacturer states that reconstituted solutions of Doxorubicin Rapid Dissolution are chemically stable for up to 48 hours at room temperature in normal artificial light.[1] Doxorubicin solution for injection, which has a pH of 3, is stable for 18 months at 2 to 8°C and for one month at room temperature.[3] A review of the literature reveals that doxorubicin appears to be chemically stable for longer periods[5–12] but data are limited and contradictory and require critical assessment.

The stability of doxorubicin depends on a number of factors, the most important of which are temperature, pH and the type of solvent used for reconstitution.[13,14] Doxorubicin is also light sensitive and adsorbs on to glass and certain plastics.

Effect of pH: Doxorubicin becomes more stable as the pH of the drug infusion fluid admixture becomes more acidic (pH 7.4 to 4.5).[6] Maximum stability is observed at about pH 4.[15]

Decomposition in acidic solution has been studied by several authors.[16,17] Acidic hydrolysis of doxorubicin (pH below 4), which is shown in Figure 1, yields a red-coloured, water-insoluble aglycone, doxorubicinone and a water-soluble amino sugar, daunosamine. Degradation follows first order kinetics.[17] The first order rate constant is directly proportional to the hydrogen ion concentration (0.01 M to 0.5 M).[16]

The rate of cleavage of the glycosidic bond, in acidic media, is strongly dependent on structural modifications in the amino sugar moiety and unaffected by structural modifications in the aglycone portion of the molecule. As doxorubicin and daunorubicin both possess daunosamine as the sugar moiety, the rate of degradation of these two analogues is similar in acidic solution.[15]

At pH values above 4, the degradation pattern of doxorubicin has not been elucidated completely. In addition to strongly alkaline solution a colour change from red to deep blue-purple is observed and rapid degradation of doxorubicin occurs. Abdeen *et al.*[18] observed that a solution of doxorubicin in 2 M sodium hydroxide was initially blue and slowly turned yellow as degradation occurred. Acidification and extraction of this mixture afforded at least five components which were not identified. Analysis of degradation mixtures at pH 8.0 by Beijnen *et al.*[15] showed one major degradation product, 7,8-dehydro-9,10-desacetyldaunorubicinone and minor quantities of other fluorescing compounds. The proposed scheme for this conversion is shown in Figure 2.

At pH values ≤9.5, degradation has been shown to be accelerated by acetate, phosphate and carbonate buffers. At pH values above 10, buffer catalysis has not been observed.[15]

In alkaline solution, the rate of degradation of the anthracyclines is affected by structural modifications in the aglycone portion of the molecule but not by structural modifications in the amino sugar moiety. As doxorubicin and epirubicin possess identical aglycones, the rate of degradation of these two analogues is similar in alkaline solution. Conversely, the rate of degradation of daunorubicin, which possesses a different aglycone, is substantially different.[15]

Effect of light: The large differences in stability which have been reported by different groups for virtually identical experiments[6,19]

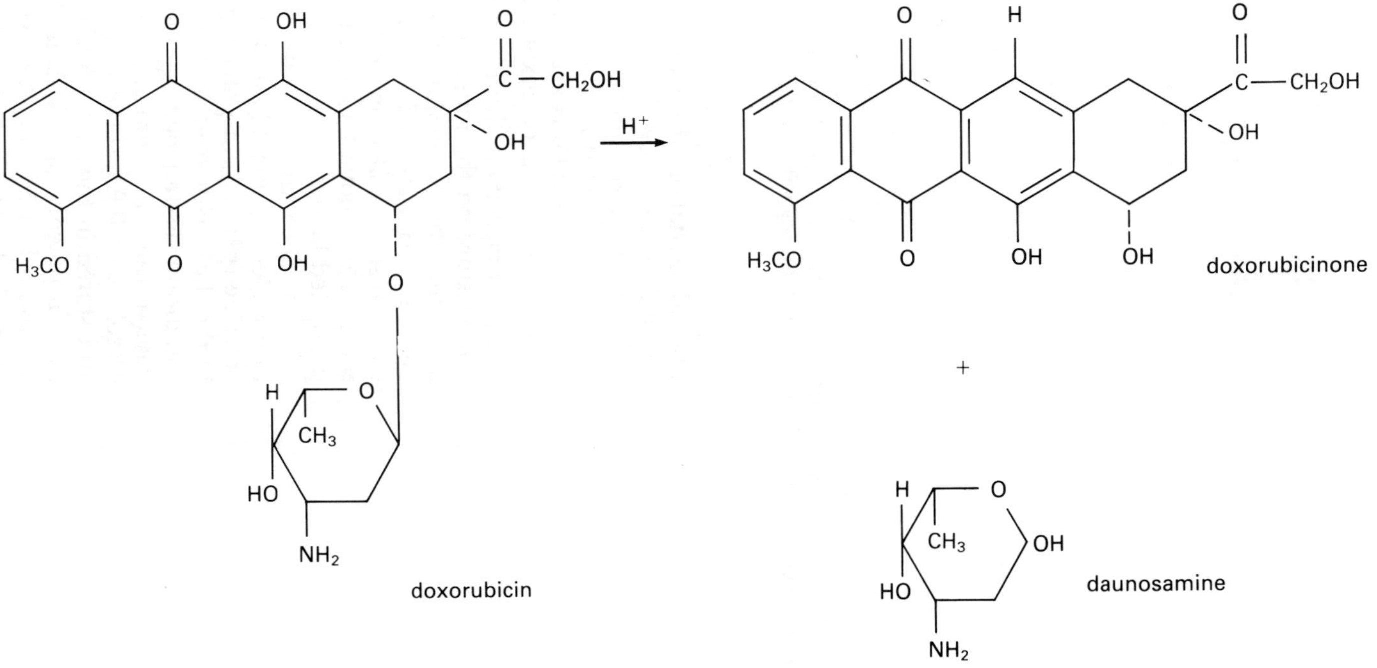

Figure 1: *Degradation pathway of doxorubicin in acidic solution*

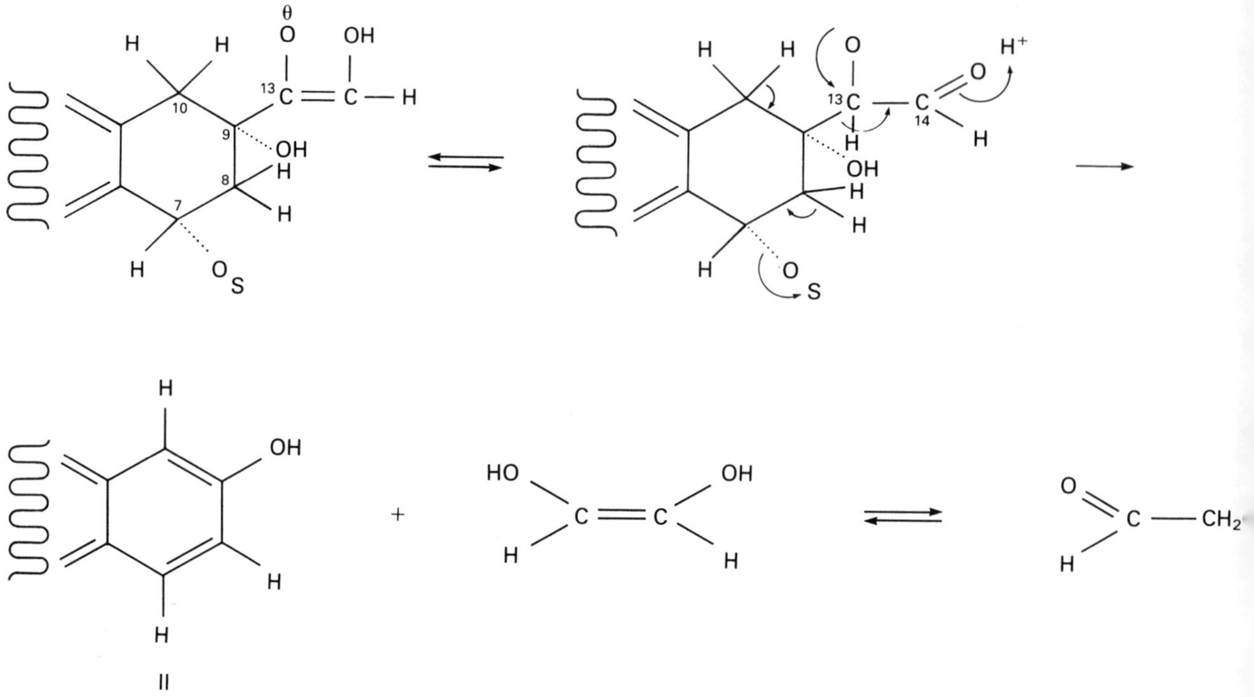

Figure 2: *Proposed degradation scheme for the conversion of doxorubicin to 7,8 dehydro-9, 10-desacetyldaunorubicinone.*[15] *S refers to the daunosamine moiety*

may be partially explained by poor control of photodegradation. Photodegradation of doxorubicin may be substantial at concentrations below 100 µg/ml, if solutions are exposed to light for sufficient time. However, at higher concentrations, such as those used for cancer chemotherapy (≥ 500 µg/ml), no special precautions are necessary to protect freshly prepared solutions of doxorubicin from light.[19,20]

Effect of temperature: Studies designed to investigate the effect of temperature on the rate of degradation of doxorubicin in buffers show that the Arrhenius relationship was obeyed for solutions between pH 4 and pH 10 between 30 and 70°C.[15] Results from stability studies at room temperature (normally 25°C), in the refrigerator (about 4°C) or in the freezer (about -20°C) are presented below.

In a well-controlled study doxorubicin was shown to be stable in 5% glucose (pH 4.7) and 3.3% glucose with 0.3% sodium chloride (pH 4.4), in polypropylene tubes, for 28 days at 25°C in the dark. However, in 0.9% sodium chloride (pH 7.0) significant degradation (greater than 10%) occurred after six days at the same temperature.[9] In another study, when dissolved in 0.9% sodium chloride (pH 6.47) in PVC minibags and stored in the dark, doxorubicin was reported to be stable (loss in potency of less than 10%) for 20 days at 25°C. In 5% glucose (pH 4.36) and 0.9% sodium chloride (pH 5.20 and pH 6.47) doxorubicin was stable in PVC minibags for at least

43 days at 4°C. In the same study, doxorubicin was also observed to be stable when reconstituted with water for injections and stored in polypropylene syringes at 4°C.[21] Finally, Hoffman *et al.*[5] observed that solutions of doxorubicin (2 mg/ml) in water for injections were stable for six months at 4°C. Those authors indicated that filtration through a 0.22 µm filter would ensure sterility without loss of drug.

Several authors have published data on the effects of freezing doxorubicin. Hoffman *et al.*[5] observed that aqueous solutions of doxorubicin (2 mg/ml) could be frozen and stored for one month at $-20°C$ without significant degradation but indicated that doxorubicin reconstituted with sodium chloride should not be frozen. Conversely, doxorubicin has been reported to be stable in 0.9% sodium chloride, for 30 days[8] and two weeks,[12] respectively, at $-20°C$. In another study, doxorubicin was reported to be stable when dissolved in 5% glucose (pH 4.36), 0.9% sodium chloride (pH 5.20 and pH 6.47) in PVC minibags for at least 43 days at $-20°C$.[21]

The effects of thawing doxorubicin by microwave radiation have also been investigated.[8,12] Karlsen *et al.*[8] observed that the concentration of doxorubicin in PVC minibags declined significantly after four re-thawings in a microwave. Keusters *et al.*[12] compared the effects of freezing and thawing doxorubicin at room temperature with thawing in the microwave. Results showed that doxorubicin was stable for two weeks at $-20°C$ when thawed by either method. After re-freezing and subsequent re-thawing a small, but significant, decrease in concentration was observed in solutions thawed by both methods. Alternatively, Hoffman *et al.*[5] observed that aqueous solutions of doxorubicin could be frozen and thawed seven times without significant loss of potency. In another study, repeated freezing and thawing of solutions of doxorubicin in PVC minibags did not lead to significant degradation.[21]

Uneven distribution of energy can occur during microwave thawing which may overheat solutions and lead to degradation.[22] For this reason, thawing in a microwave is not recommended. If frozen, doxorubicin should be thawed at room temperature.

Container compatibility: Doxorubicin is compatible with polypropylene, polyethylene, PVC and glass.[21] It has been reported to be more stable in plastic (PVC) than glass.[7] Doxorubicin adsorbs on to glass and polyethylene but not on to siliconized glass or polypropylene.[10] Solutions which contain concentrations of 2 mg/ml do not adsorb to membrane filters but, with more dilute solutions especially when associated with small volumes, greater than 95% of doxorubicin adsorbs to cellulose ester membranes and about 40% binds to polytetrafluoroethylene (PTFE) membranes.[23,24] In clinical practice, when doxorubicin is used at concentrations of at least 500 µg/ml, adsorption during storage and delivery is negligible.[21]

Compatibility with other drugs: Doxorubicin is incompatible with heparin, dexamethasone sodium phosphate, hydrocortisone sodium succinate and diazepam as precipitation occurs.[1] The manufacturers recommend that no other drugs are mixed with doxorubicin. Combinations of doxorubicin and fluorouracil or aminophylline result in a colour change from red to blue-purple which indicates the onset of rapid degradation of doxorubicin.[25]

A combination of doxorubicin and vincristine in 0.9% sodium chloride and in a mixture of 2.5% glucose with 0.45% sodium chloride, appears to be stable for at least seven days.[26] A mixture of doxorubicin and vinblastine in 0.9% sodium chloride appears to be relatively stable for at least five days.[27] The manufacturer recommends that doxorubicin is not mixed with other drugs.[1]

Stability in clinical practice

Doxorubicin is compatible with polypropylene, polyethylene, PVC and glass.[21] Doxorubicin appears to be chemically stable in PVC minibags for at least 28 days in 5% glucose or 0.9% sodium chloride when stored at 4°C and −20°C, and in polypropylene syringes for at least 28 days at 4°C.

4 Clinical Use

Main indications: Successfully used to produce regression in acute leukaemia, lymphomas, soft tissue and osteogenic sarcomas, paediatric malignancies and adult solid tumours, especially breast and lung carcinomas. Doxorubicin is frequently used in combination regimens with other cytotoxics.[1]

Dosage: Dosage is usually calculated on the basis of body surface area. For single agent therapy, 60 to 70 mg/m^2 is given every three weeks. When administered in combination with other agents which possess overlapping toxicity, dosage may need to be reduced to 30 to 40 mg/m^2 every three weeks. If the dosage is to be calculated on the basis of body weight, 1.2 to 2.4 mg/kg is given as a single dose every three weeks. The total dose for the cycle may be divided over three successive days (20 to 25 mg/m^2 on each day). Administration of doxorubicin on a weekly regimen (20 mg/m^2) has been shown to be as effective as the three-weekly regimen. Dosage may need to be reduced in patients who have had prior treatment with other cytotoxics, in children and the elderly. If hepatic function is impaired, doxorubicin dosage should be reduced to 50% of the normal dose when serum bilirubin concentrations are 1.2 to >3 mg/100 ml, and to 25% of the normal dose when serum bilirubin concentrations are more than 3 mg/100 ml.

A cumulative dose of 450 mg to 550 mg/m^2 should only be exceeded with extreme caution as the risk of irreversible congestive cardiac failure increases greatly.[1]

5 Preparation of Injection

Reconstitution: The contents of the 10 mg vial are reconstituted with 5 ml of water for injections or 0.9% sodium chloride, the

20 mg vial with 10 ml and the 50 mg vial with 25 ml of the same solvent. After addition of the diluent, the contents of the vial will dissolve within 30 seconds, with gentle shaking and without inversion, to produce a solution of 2 mg/ml.[1]

Bolus administration: Administration is most frequently by the intravenous route. The manufacturer recommends that the reconstituted solution is given over two to three minutes, via the tubing of a freely-running intravenous infusion of 0.9% sodium chloride, 5% glucose or sodium chloride with glucose. This technique minimizes the risk of thrombosis or perivenous extravasation which can lead to severe cellulitis or vesication. Doxorubicin may also be administered by the intra-arterial or intravesical route.[1]

Infusion: Although the optimum schedule of continuous infusion of doxorubicin has not been established, most current investigations can be grouped into two broad categories. Most experience has been acquired using a schedule of short-term infusions given over one to four days, with cycles repeated every three to four weeks. The most thoroughly investigated short-term infusion has been the 96-hour cycle which generally takes five days to complete. In more recent studies, patients have received infusions for several months or longer.

Based on the marked decrease in the cardiac toxicity seen with short-term infusions of doxorubicin, a number of investigators have recently initiated studies with low dose doxorubicin given as a continuous infusion on a more protracted basis.[28–31] Starting with a daily dose of 1 to 2 mg/m^2 the maximum total daily dose has varied between 3 and 5 mg/m^2 for periods of several weeks to several months in responding patients. Some investigators have used higher daily doses for two-week cycles of therapy followed by two weeks without chemotherapy to allow for recovery from side-effects.[32]

Gloves for handling: Rubber gloves are recommended.

Extravasation: Doxorubicin is a potent vesicant. Care should be taken to avoid extravasation during intravenous infusion. Should extravasation occur the infusion should be stopped immediately and resumed in another vein. Appropriate treatment for the extravasated area should be commenced immediately.

6 Destruction of Drug or Contaminated Articles

Incineration: 700°C.[3]

Chemical: Dilute sodium hypochlorite (1% available chlorine)/ 24 hours.[1]

Contact with skin: Wash with water, soap and water, or sodium bicarbonate solution. If the eyes are contaminated immediate irrigation with saline should be carried out.[1]

References

1. ABPI Data Sheet Compendium 1989/1990. (1989). Datapharm Publications Ltd, London, pp. 465–467.

2. Doxorubicin Solution for Injection. Data sheet. (1989). Farmitalia Carlo Erba Ltd, St Albans, Herts, UK.

3. Personal communication, Farmitalia Carlo Erba Ltd. Unpublished data.

4. Anon. (1989). *The Extra Pharmacopoeia*, 29th edn, Reynolds J.E.F. (ed.), Pharmaceutical Press, London, pp. 623–626.

5. Hoffman, D.M. *et al.* (1979). Stability of refrigerated and frozen solutions of doxorubicin hydrochloride. *Am. J. Hosp. Pharm.* **36**, 1536–1538.

6. Poochikian, G.K. *et al.* (1981). Stability of anthracycline antitumour agents in four infusion fluids. *Am. J. Hosp. Pharm.* **38**, 483–486.

7. Benvenuto, J.A. *et al.* (1981). Stability and compatibility of antitumour agents in glass and plastic containers. *Am. J. Hosp. Pharm.* **38**, 1914–1918.

8. Karlsen, J. *et al.* (1983). Stability of cytotoxic intravenous solutions subjected to freeze-thaw treatment. *Nor. Pharm. Acta.* **45**, 61–67.

9. Beijnen, J.H. *et al.* (1985a). Stability of anthracycline antitumour agents in infusion fluids. *J. Parent. Sci. Technol.* **39**, 220–222.

10. Bosanquet, A.G. (1986). Stability of solutions of antineoplastic agents during preparation and storage for *in vitro* assays. II. Assay methods, Adriamycin and the other antitimour antibiotics. *Cancer Chemother. Pharmacol.* **17**, 1–10.

11. Bouma, J. *et al.* (1986). Anthracycline antitumour agents: A review of physicochemical, analytical and stability properties. *Pharm. Weekbl. (Sci. edn)* **8**, 109–135.

12. Keusters, L. *et al.* (1986). Stability of solutions of doxorubicin and epirubicin in plastic minibags for intravesical use after storage at −20°C and thawing by microwave radiation. *Pharm. Weekbl. (Sci. edn)* **8**, 194–197.

13. Gupta, P.K. *et al.* (1988). Investigation of the stability of doxorubicin hydrochloride using factorial design. *Drug Develop. Indust. Pharm.* **14**, 1657–1671.

14. Janssen, M.J.H. *et al.* (1985). Doxorubicin decomposition on storage: Effect of pH, type of buffer and liposome encapsulation. *Int. J. Pharm.* **23**, 1–11.

15. Beijnen, J.H. *et al.* (1968a). Aspects of the degradation kinetics of doxorubicin in aqueous solution. *Int. J. Pharm.* **32**, 123–131.

16. Wasserman, K. and Bundgaard, H. (1983). Kinetics of the acid catalysed hydrolysis of doxorubicin. *Int. J. Pharm.* **14**, 73–78.

17. Beijnen, J.H. *et al.* (1985b). Aspects of the stability of doxorubicin and seven other anthracyclines in acidic solution. *Pharm. Weekbl. (Sci. edn)* **7**, 109–116.

18. Abdeen, Z. *et al.* (1985). Degradation of Adriamycin in aqueous sodium hydroxide: Formation of a ring-A oxabicyclononenone. *J. Chem. Research (S)* 254–255.

19. Tavoloni, N. *et al.* (1980). Photolytic degradation of Adriamycin. Communications: *J. Pharm. Pharmacol.* **32**, 860–862.

20. Wood, M.J. *et al.* (1990) Photodegradation of doxorubicin, daunorubicin and epirubicin measured by high-performance liquid chromatography. *J. Clin. Pharm. Ther.* (In Press).
21. Wood, M.J. *et al.* (1990). Stability of doxorubicin, daunorubicin and epirubicin in plastic syringes and minibags. *J. Clin. Pharm. Ther.* (In Press).
22. Williamson, M. and Luce, J.K. (1987). Microwave thawing of doxorubicin hydrochloride admixtures not recommended. *Am. J. Hosp. Pharm.* **44**, 505 and 510.
23. Pavlik, E.J. *et al.* (1982). Sensitivity of anticancer agents *in vitro*, standardizing the cytotoxic response and characterizing the sensitivities of a reference cell line. *Gynecol. Oncol.* **14**, 243–261.
24. Pavlik, E.J. *et al.* (1984). Stability of doxorubicin in relation to chemosensitivity determinations: loss of lethality and retention of antiproliferative activity. *Cancer Invest.* **2**, 449–458.
25. Trissel, L.A. (1988). *Handbook of injectable drugs*, 5th edn, American Society of Hospital Pharmacists, Bethesda, Maryland, USA.
26. Beijnen, J.H. *et al.* (1986b). Stability of intravenous admixtures of doxorubicin and vincristine. *Am. J. Hosp. Pharm.* **43**, 3022–3027.
27. Gaj, E. and Sesin, P. (1984). Compatibility of doxorubicin hydrochloride and vinblastine sulphate. The stability of a solution stored in Cormed reservoir bags or Monoject plastic syringes. *Am. J. Intraven. Therap. Clin. Nutrit.* **11**, 8–20.
28. Garnick, M.B. *et al.* (1983). Clinical evaluation of long-term continuous infusion doxorubicin. *Cancer Treat. Reports* **67**, 133–142.
29. Bowen, J. *et al.* (1981). Phase I study of Adriamycin by 5-day continuous intravenous infusion. *Proc. Am. Assoc. Cancer Res.*, **22**, 354 (C-84).
30. Lokich, J.J. *et al.* (1983) Constant infusion schedule for Adriamycin: A phase I–II clinical trial of a 30-day schedule by ambulatory pump delivery system. *J. Clin. Oncol.* **1**, 24–28.
31. Vogelsang, W.J. *et al.* (1984). Continuous doxorubicin infusion using an implanted lithium battery-powered drug administration device system (DADS, Medtronic, Inc.).*Proc. Am. Soc. Clin. Oncol.* **3**, 263 (C-1030).
32. Legha, S.S. *et al.* (1987). Anthracyclines: In Cancer chemotherapy by infusion, Lokich J.J. (ed.). MTP Press Ltd, London.

Prepared by M.J. Wood

EPIRUBICIN

1 General Details

Approved name: Epirubicin.

Proprietary name: Pharmorubicin.

Manufacturer or supplier: Farmitalia Carlo Erba Ltd.

Presentation and formulation details: Sterile, pyrogen-free, red, freeze-dried powder in vials containing 10 mg, 20 mg and 50 mg of epirubicin hydrochloride with lactose. There are no preservatives in the preparation.[1]

Storage and shelf-life of unopened container: Dry unopened vials expire three years from the date of manufacture when stored in a dry place protected from sunlight. Vials of epirubicin are stored at room temperature.[1]

2 Chemistry

Type: A cytotoxic antibiotic consisting of an amino sugar, acosamine, linked through a glycosidic bond to the C7 of a tetracyclic aglycone, doxorubicinone.

Molecular structure:

Molecular weight: 580.0.

Solubility: Epirubicin is soluble in water for injections, 5% glucose and 0.9% sodium chloride, partially soluble in methanol and ethanol and practically insoluble in chloroform, ether and other organic solvents.[2]

3 Stability Profile

Physical and chemical stability

The manufacturer states that the reconstituted solution is chemically stable for up to 48 hours at 2 to 8°C or 24 hours at room temperature.[1] The literature indicates that epirubicin may be chemically stable for longer periods, although little data has been published.[3,4]

The stability of epirubicin depends on a number of factors. Degradation in aqueous solution is pH dependent. Epirubicin is also light sensitive and adsorbs to glass and certain plastics.

Effect of pH: Acidic hydrolysis of epirubicin (pH below 4.0), shown in Figure 1, yields a red-coloured, water-insoluble aglycone, doxorubicinone, and a water-soluble amino sugar,

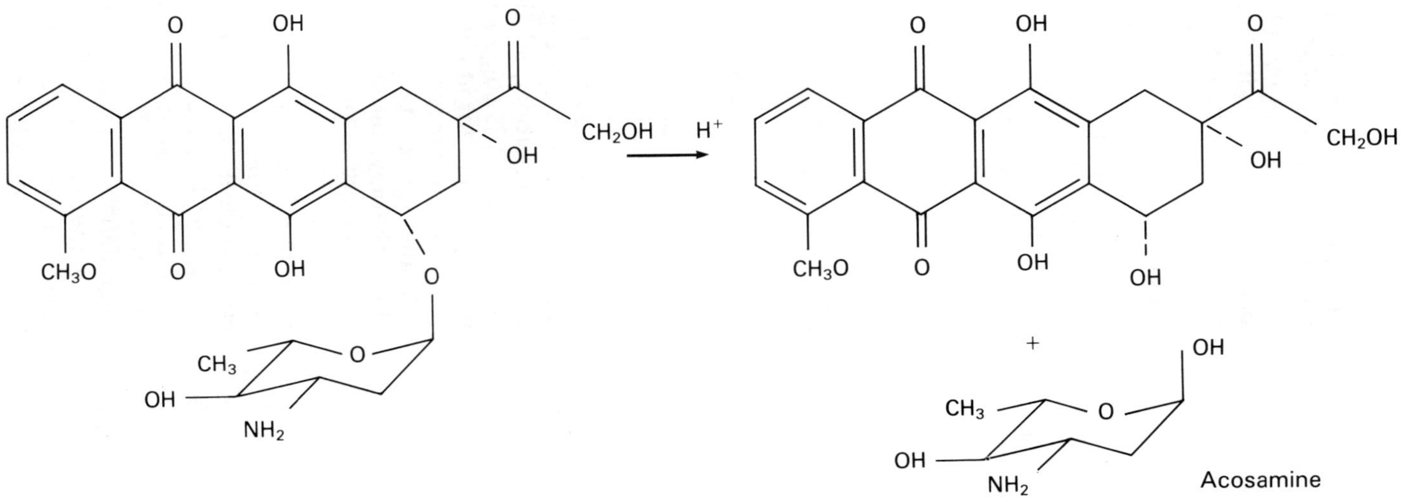

Figure 1: *Degradation pathway of epirubicin in acidic solution*

acosamine. The rate of cleavage of the glycosidic bond in acidic media is strongly affected by structural differences in the amino sugar moiety and unaffected by structural differences in the aglycone portion of the molecule. As doxorubicin and epirubicin possess different amino sugar residues, the rate of degradation of these two analogues in acidic solution is different.[5]

At pH values above 4.0, the degradation pathway of epirubicin has not been elucidated. However, on addition to strongly alkaline solution a colour change from red to deep blue-purple is observed and rapid degradation occurs. Data on the degradation of epirubicin in alkaline solution have recently been published, indicating that, at pH 8.0, the main degradation product is 7,8,-dehydro-9,10-desacetyldaunorubicinone.[5] The structure of this compound is shown in Figure 2.

In alkaline solution the rate of degradation of the anthracyclines is affected by structural differences in the aglycone portion of the molecule and unaffected by structural differences in the amino sugar moiety. As epirubicin and doxorubicin possess the same aglycone, their rates of degradation in alkaline solution are similar.[5]

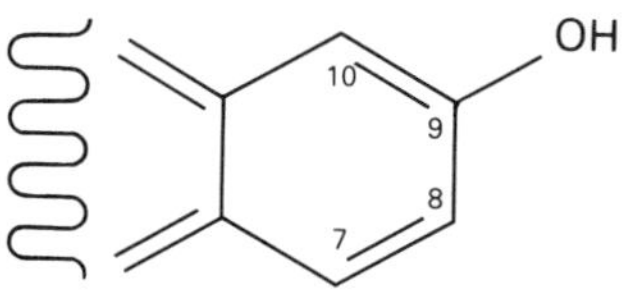

Figure 2:   *Structure of 7,8,-dehydro-9,10-desacetyldaunorubicinone[5]*

Effect of light: Data on the kinetics of degradation of doxorubicin in fluorescent light have been published[6] but, until recently, there were no data available for epirubicin. Results from a study in which the rates of photodegradation of doxorubicin, daunorubicin and epirubicin were compared indicated that the rate of photodegradation of epirubicin was similar to doxorubicin. This suggests that photodegradation of epirubicin may be significant at concentrations below 100 µg/ml if solutions are exposed to light for sufficient time.[7] However, at higher concentrations, such as those used for cancer chemotherapy, (at least 500 µg/ml), no special precautions are necessary to protect freshly prepared solutions of epirubicin from light.[7]

Effect of temperature: Little data has been published on the effect of temperature on the stability of epirubicin. In a well-controlled study, epirubicin was shown to be stable, in polypropylene tubes, in 5% glucose (pH 4.7) and 3.3% glucose with 0.3% sodium chloride (pH 4.4) for 28 days at 25°C, when stored in the dark. However, in 0.9% sodium chloride (pH 7.0) significant degradation occurred after eight days at the same temperature.[3] In another study, epirubicin was reported to be stable for at least 43 days in PVC minibags in 5% glucose (pH 4.36) and 0.9% sodium chloride (pH 5.20) at 25°C.[8] However, when dissolved in 0.9% sodium chloride (pH 6.47), epirubicin was only stable for 24 days at the same temperature. In the same study, epirubicin was reported to be stable for at least 43 days, when reconstituted with water for injections and stored in polypropylene syringes at 4°C.[8]

There are two studies which have investigated the effects of freezing epirubicin. In the first, epirubicin was reported to be stable for four weeks when frozen at −20°C in PVC minibags containing 0.9% sodium chloride.[4] In the second, epirubicin was observed to be stable for at least 43 days in PVC minibags containing 5% glucose (pH 4.36) and 0.9% sodium chloride (pH 5.20 and 6.47) at −20°C.[8] Repeated freezing and re-thawing these minibags at ambient temperature did not cause degradation[8]

Container compatibility: Epirubicin is compatible with polypropylene, PVC and glass.[8] Epirubicin adsorbs on to glass and polyethylene but not to siliconized glass or polypropylene.[8] However, in clinical practice, when epirubicin is used at concentrations of at least 500 µg/ml, adsorptive losses during storage and delivery are negligible.[8]

Compatibility with other drugs: Epirubicin should not be mixed with heparin as a precipitate may form.[1] The manufacturers recommend that epirubicin is not mixed with any other drugs.

Stability in clinical practice

Epirubicin is compatible with polypropylene, PVC and glass.[8] Epirubicin appears to be chemically stable in PVC minibags for at least 28 days in 5% glucose and 0.9% sodium chloride at 4°C and −20°C, and in polypropylene syringes for at least 28 days at 4°C.[8] After reconstitution, vials of epirubicin (2 mg/ml) are stable for at least 14 days at 4°C.[8]

4 Clinical Use

Main indications: Epirubicin as a single agent has produced regression in a wide range of neoplastic conditions including breast, ovarian, gastric and colorectal carcinomas, lymphomas, leukaemias and multiple myeloma. Epirubicin may be used in combination with other cytotoxic agents.[1]

Dosage and administration: Dosage is usually calculated on the basis of body surface area. For single agent therapy the dose range most commonly used is 75 to 90 mg/m^2 every three weeks. The total dose for the cycle may be divided over two successive days. When epirubicin is used in combination therapy with other cytotoxics the dosage should be reduced. Dosage should also be reduced in hepatic impairment.[1]

Epirubicin can be administered on a weekly regimen, particularly for the palliative treatment of poor-risk patients for whom the toxicity of a conventional three-weekly regimen would be unacceptable. For these patients, the most commonly used dose is 20 mg per week. A cumulative dose of 700 mg/m^2 should only be exceeded with extreme caution as the risk of irreversible congestive cardiac failure increases greatly.[1]

5 Preparation of Injection

Reconstitution: The contents of the 10 mg vial are reconstituted with 5 ml of water for injections, the 20 mg vial with 10 ml, and the 50 mg vial with 25 ml of the same solvent. After addition of the diluent and gentle shaking the contents of the vial will dissolve to produce a solution of 2 mg/ml. Reconstitution may occasionally result in the formation of a gelatinous mass which will redissolve completely on further shaking.[1]

Bolus administration: Administration is licensed only by the intravenous route. The reconstituted solution is given, over three to five minutes, via the tubing of a freely-running intravenous infusion of 0.9% sodium chloride. This technique minimizes the risk of thrombosis or perivenous extravasation, which can lead to severe cellulitis or vesication. Administration of epirubicin by intravesical, intra-arterial, intrapleural and intraperitoneal routes has been investigated in clinical trials.[9–11]

Infusion: Continuous infusion schedules of epirubicin have been investigated in the USA. At New York University, epirubicin has been given as a six hour infusion.[12] At MD Anderson Memorial Hospital, a 48-hour infusion of doxorubicin (60 to 70 mg/m^2) has been compared with a 48-hour infusion of epirubicin (90 to 105 mg/m^2).[13]

Gloves for handling: Rubber gloves are recommended.

Extravasation: Epirubicin is a potent vesicant. Care should be taken to avoid extravasation during intravenous administration. Should extravasation occur, the infusion should be stopped immediately and resumed in another vein. Appropriate treatment for the extravasated area should be commenced immediately.

6 Destruction of Drug or Contaminated Articles

Incineration: 700°C.[14]

Chemical: Dilute sodium hypochlorite (1% available chlorine)/ 24 hours.[1]

Contact with skin: Wash with water, soap and water, or sodium bicarbonate solution. If the eyes are contaminated, immediate irrigation with saline should be carried out.[1]

References

1. ABPI Data Sheet Compendium 1989/1990. (1989). Datapharm Publications Ltd, London, pp. 473–475.
2. Anon. (1989). *The Extra Pharmacopoeia.* 29th edn, Reynolds, J.E.F. (ed.), Pharmaceutical Press, London, p. 626.

3. Beijnen, J.H. *et al.* (1985). Stability of anthracycline antitumour agents in infusion fluids. *J. Parent. Sci. Technol.* **39**, 220–222.
4. Keusters, L. *et al.* (1986). Stability of solutions of doxorubicin and epirubicin in plastic minibags for intravesical use after storage at −20°C and thawing by microwave radiation. *Pharm. Weekbl. (Sci. edn)* **8**, 194–197.
5. Beijnen, J.H. *et al.* (1986) Aspects of the degradation kinetics of doxorubicin in aqueous solution. *Int. J. Pharm.* **32**, 123–131.
6. Tavoloni, N. *et al.* (1980). Photolytic degradation of Adriamycin. Communications: *J. Pharm. Pharmacol.* **32**, 860–862.
7. Wood, M.J. *et al.* (1990). Photodegradation of doxorubicin, daunorubicin and epirubicin measured by high-performance liquid chromatography. *J. Clin. Pharm. Ther.* (In Press).
8. Wood, M.J. *et al.* (1990). Stability of doxorubicin, daunorubicin and epirubicin in plastic syringes and minibags. *J. Clin. Pharm. Ther.* (In Press).
9. Ferrazzi, E. *et al.* (1982). Preliminary phase II experience with 4′epidoxorubicin: In *Anthracycline antibiotics in cancer therapy*. Muggia, F.M., Young, C.W., Carter, S.K. (eds), Martinus Nijhoff, The Hague, p. 562.
10. Strocchi, E. *et al.* (1983). 4′epidoxorubicin in locoregional therapy: Pharmacokinetic study after intrahepatic arterial and intraperitoneal administration. Proc. 4th NCI-EORTC Symposium, Brussels (Abst. 108).
11. Friedman, M.A. and Ignoffo, R.J. (1984). Intra-arterial use of adriamycin: In *Adriamycin: Its expanding role in cancer treatment*. Ogawa, M., Muggia, F.M., Rozencweig, M. (eds), Excerpta Medica, Tokyo, p. 387.
12. Muggia, F.M. and Green, M.D. (1984). Special modes of administration: In *Advances in anthracycline chemotherapy: Epirubicin*. Bonnadonna, G. (ed.), Milano, pp. 149–152.
13. Bodey, G.P. *et al.* (1983). Clinical trials with 4′epidoxorubicin. Proc. 13th International Congress of Chemotherapy, Vienna, part 215/23, Masson, Canada.
14. Personal communication, Farmitalia Carlo Erba Ltd. Unpublished data.

Prepared by M.J. Wood

ETHOGLUCID

1 General Details

Approved names: Etoglucid, Ethoglucid.

Proprietary name: Epodyl.

Manufacturer: ICI Pharmaceuticals Ltd.

Presentation and formulation details: Ampoules containing 1 ml (1.13 g) liquid ethoglucid.

Storage and shelf-life of unopened containers: Four years when stored at room temperature.

2 Chemistry

Type: Alkylating agent.

Molecular weight: 262.3.

Molecular structure: 2,2'-(2,5,8,11-tetraoxadodecane-1,12-diyl) bis-oxirane

$$CH_2\text{-}CH\text{-}CH_2\text{-}O\text{-}CH_2\text{-}CH_2\text{-}O\text{-}CH_2\text{-}CH_2\text{-}O\text{-}CH_2\text{-}CH_2\text{-}O\text{-}CH_2\text{-}CH\text{-}CH_2$$

Solubility: Miscible in all proportions with water.

3 Stability Profile

Physical and chemical stability

Ethoglucid is hydrolysed in aqueous solution, the epoxide ring being opened to form the 1,2 and 15,16 diols. Epoxide hydrolysis is acid- and base-catalyzed, so ethoglucid would be expected to be less stable in acid or alkaline conditions than in neutral solution.

Ethoglucid is not especially sensitive to light and no particular precautions are required.

Container compatibility: Ethoglucid is not absorbed from solutions in polypropylene syringes or PVC bags. Studies on 1% solutions in three brands of polypropylene syringes, and 1% and 2% solutions in PVC bags have shown that observed drug losses are due to hydrolytic degradation and not absorption.[1]

Stability in clinical practice

Ethoglucid is administered as a 1% or 2% solution in water for injections or normal saline. Solutions are stable for 14 days at 4°C, two days at room temperature and 16 hours at 37°C.[1] The anti-tumour acitivty is unaffected by changes in urine osmolarity[2] or pH[3].

4 Clinical Use

Type of cytotoxic agent: Alkylating agent.

Main indications: Ethoglucid is used for the treatment of non-invasive tumours of the bladder.

Dosage: By instillation, as a 1% or 2% v/v solution of ethoglucid in water for injections or normal saline. Treatment may be repeated daily for two weeks, then at less frequent intervals.

5 Preparation of Solutions

Dilution: The contents of an ampoule are added to 50 or 100 ml water for injections or normal saline to give a 2% or 1% solution, respectively.

Gloves for handling: PVC gloves recommended.

Administration: The solution should be instilled into the bladder and retained there as long as possible. The patient's fluid intake should be restricted beforehand.

6 Destruction of Drug or Contaminated Articles

Incineration: 1100°C.

Chemical: Add one volume of concentrated hydrochloric acid to three volumes ethoglucid solution and allow to react for 30 minutes. Neutralize the resultant solution with sodium hydroxide and discard to drain.[4]

Contact with skin: Wash with water.

References

1. Lee, M.G. (1985). Stability of ethoglucid bladder irrigation in plastics. *Pharm. J.* **235**, 653.
2. Groos, E. and Masters, J.R.W. (1986). Intravesical chemotherapy: Studies on the relationships between osmolarity and cytotoxicity. *J. Urol.* **136**, 399–402.
3. Groos, E. *et al.* (1986). Intravesical chemotherapy. Studies on the relationships between pH and cytotoxicity. *Cancer,* **58**, 1199–1203.
4. Wilson, V.J. (1983). Safe disposal of some commonly used injectable antineoplastic drugs. *J. Clin. Hosp. Pharm.* **8**, 295–299.

Prepared by M.G. Lee

ETOPOSIDE

1 General Details

Approved name: Etoposide.

Proprietary name: Vepesid.

Manufacturer or supplier: Bristol-Myers Co. Ltd and E R Squibb & Sons.

Presentation and formulation details: Glass ampoules containing 100 mg etoposide in 5 ml solution.

Each ml contains:

etopside	20 mg
polyethylene glycol 300	650 mg
ethylalcohol	241 mg
polysorbate 80	80 mg
benzyl alcohol	30 mg
citric acid	2 mg

Storage and shelf-life of unopened container: Five years from the date of manufacture when stored at room temperature and protected from light.

2 Chemistry

Type: Semi-synthetic podophyllotoxin derivative.

Molecular structure: 4-0-Demethyl-1-1 0-(4,6-0-Ethylidene-β-D-glucopyranosyl)epi-podophyllotoxin.

Molecular weight: 588.6.

Solubility: Highly insoluble in water,[6] soluble in organic solvents.[2] In dilutions with 0.9% sodium chloride, the concentration of etoposide should not exceed 0.25 mg/ml,[1] although it is suggested concentrations up to 0.4 mg/ml are acceptable.[6]

3 Stability Profile

Physical and chemical stability

Etoposide degrades by hydrolytic cleavage of the glycopyranoxyl moiety.

Effect of pH: No information available.

Effect of light: Etoposide should be protected from light during storage[1] and from strong daylight during administration.

Container compatibility: Glass or PVC containers are recommended,[1] and polypropylene syringes are also acceptable.[5,6] Etoposide is incompatible with cellulose acetate membrane filters but compatible with nylon or fluripore type membranes.[9] Undiluted etoposide injection has been implicated in the formation of hairline cracks in infusion devices constructed of plastics produced from the monomers acrylonitrile, butadiene and styrene.[10] The effect on these plastics (known collectively as ABS plastic) has been attributed to the action of polyethylene glycol (PEG) 300, a solubilizing agent in the injectable formulation. Caution should be exercised in the use of any plastic infusion device with undiluted etoposide injection.

Compatibility with other drugs: 5% glucose and 0.9% sodium chloride are recommended as diluents for the infusion of etoposide.[7] The manufacturer does not recommend mixing etoposide with any other drug.[1]

Stability in clinical practice

At concentrations of 0.2 and 0.4 mg/ml in 5% glucose and in 0.9% sodium chloride, the solutions are stable for 96 and 48 hours respectively at 25°C in normal fluorescent lighting before precipitation occurs.[3] However, other studies[4] suggested that the drug may be daylight-sensitive and is unstable beyond six hours in unprotected solutions.

Etoposide infusions (0.2 mg/ml) in PVC containers of sodium chloride 0.9% or 5% glucose exhibited no loss of etoposide over 72 hours storage at 5 or 25°C.[5] It was concluded from this study that etoposide was not adsorbed on to the surface of the container. Polypropylene syringes containing etoposide infusion (1 mg/ml in water for injections) prepared for continuous infusion were chemically stable at 4 and 20°C for 28 days.[6] However, as precipitation of etoposide during administration was found to occur, great care is necessary.

4 Clinical Use

Type of cytotoxic agent: Mitotic inhibitor which arrests the cell cycle in the G2 phase.

Main indications: Small cell carcinoma of the lung. Resistant non-seminomatous testicular carcinoma.

Dosage by injection: 60 to 120 mg/m² by IV infusion daily, for five consecutive days repeated every three to four weeks. Alternatively, 100 mg/m² day on days 1, 2, 3, 5 every three to four weeks.

Oral: Twice the IV dose should be given on five consecutive days every three to four weeks, myelosuppression permitting.

5 Preparation of the Injection

Dilution: The injection should be diluted in 5% glucose or 0.9% sodium chloride solution to give a concentration of 0.25 mg/ml etoposide in the infusion.

Bolus administration: Not recommended.

Infusion administration: The dose should be given by IV infusion over not less than 30 minutes.

Gloves for handling: Rubber gloves of surgical thickness.[8]

Extravasation: Mildly irritant. Elevate the limb, pack the surrounding area with ice, administer local hydrocortisone to the affected area and needle aspirate any obvious fluid swelling.

6 Destruction of Drug or Contaminated Articles

Incineration: 1000°C.

Chemical: 5% sodium hypochlorite solution 24 hours.

Contact with skin: Accidental exposure to etoposide may cause skin reactions. A soap and water wash should be employed.

References

1. ABPI Data Sheet Compendium 1989/90. (1989). Datapharm Publications Ltd, London, pp. 261–262.
2. Anon. (1982). *The Extra Pharmacopoeia*, 29th edn, Reynolds, J.E.F. (ed.), Pharmaceutical Press, London, pp. 208–209.
3. Phillips, N.C. and Lauper, R.D. (1983). Review of etoposide. *Clin. Pharm.* **2**, 112–119.
4. Arnold, A.M. (1979). Podophyllotoxin derivative VP 16–213. *Cancer Chemother. Pharmacol.* **3**, 71–80.
5. Sewell, G.J. (1988). Adsorption of etoposide (Vepesid) on to PVC of Viaflex infusion bags. Unpublished report, No. 67.
6. Adams, P.S. *et al.* (1987). Pharmaceutical aspects of home infusion therapy for cancer patients. *Pharm. J.* **238**, 476–478.
7. Trissel, L.A. (1988) *Handbook on injectable drugs*, 5th edn. American Society of Hospital Pharmacists, Bethesda, Maryland, USA.
8. Laidlaw, J.A. *et al.* (1984). Permeability of latex and PVC gloves to 20 antineoplastic drugs. *Am. J. Hosp. Pharm.* **41**, 2618–2623.
9. Forrest, S.C. (1984). Vepesid Injection, *Pharm J.* **232**, 88.
10. Schwinghammer, T.L. and Reilly, M. (1988). Cracking of ABS plastic devices used to infuse undiluted etoposide injection (letter). *Am. J. Hosp. Pharm.* **45**, 1277.

Prepared by G.J. Sewell

FLUOROURACIL

1 General Details

Approved names: Fluorouracil, 5-fluorouracil.

Proprietary names: Fluoro-uracil, Efudix.

Manufacturer or suppliers: Roche Products Ltd, David Bull Laboratories Ltd (DBL).

Presentation and formulation details: Colourless to slightly yellow solution in clear glass ampoules (Roche) or rubber-capped clear glass vials (DBL) containing 25 mg/ml fluorouracil; solution in water for injections with sodium hydroxide for pH adjustment.

Storage and shelf-life of unopened container: The shelf-life is two years when stored at room temperature and protected from light.

2 Chemistry

Type: Fluorinated pyrimidine.

Molecular structure: 5-Fluoro-2,4(1H,3H)pyrimidine-dione.

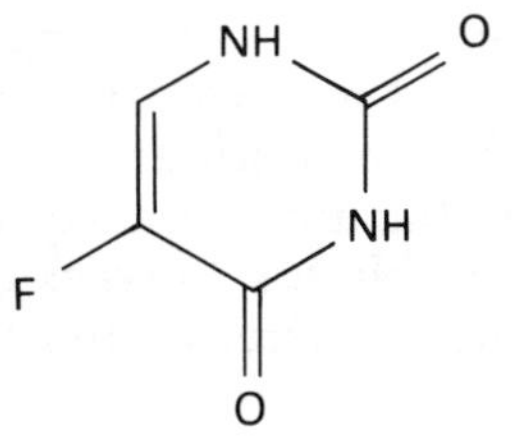

Molecular weight: 130.1.

Solubility: 12.5 mg/ml in water; 6 mg/ml in ethanol.

3 Stability Profile

Physical and chemical stability

Fluorouracil breakdown occurs by two routes: thermal and photochemical decomposition cause the opening of the pyrimidine ring between N3 and C4 and N1 and C5 to produce urea. Alkaline hydrolysis leads to the production of barbituric acid and uracil which further degrades to urea. The rate of alkaline hydrolysis increases rapidly above pH 9.0 so the injection is formulated within the pH range of 8.6 to 9.0. Although the drug is stable at acid pH, solubility is reduced.

The injection should be protected from strong daylight and temperatures above 25°C.

Container compatibility: Many studies has been made of container compatibility at various concentrations. At concentrations of 5 to 10 mg/ml, the drug has been shown to be stable for 16 weeks at 5°C in PVC containers. Similar and more concentrated solutions have been shown to be stable for up to 42 days at room temperature.[1,2,3] A small increase in concentration resulted from loss of moisture. Undiluted injections have been stored in a plastic syringe or glass vial without loss of potency.[4] Studies for the Exeter continuous chemotherapy infusion programme have shown the undiluted injection to be stable for 28 days at 5°C and 25°C in plastic syringes.[5]

Compatibility with other drugs: Compatible with 5% glucose,[1,6,7] bleomycin,[8] prednisolone sodium phosphate, vincristine sulphate[9] and calcium leucovorin.[10] It is also compatible with methotrexate and cyclophosphamide.[11] Fluorouracil is incompatible with acidic drugs or drugs that decompose in an alkaline environment, eg doxorubicin,[12] it is also compatible with cytarabine,[9] and diazepam.[12] McRae and King[9] found that fluorouracil is incompatible with methotrexate, although this is contradicted by Lokich *et al.*[11]

Stability in clinical practice

The drug has been shown to be quite stable at pH values below 9.0 and when protected from strong daylight and temperatures above 25°C. In syringes and PVC containers, undiluted or diluted in 0.9% sodium chloride, the drug has been shown to be stable for at least 28 days. In 5% glucose, there is some conflicting evidence. One study has indicated that the drug is stable for 16 weeks at 5°C[1] or five days at room temperature,[6] whereas other workers reported a loss of 10% in 43 hours.[7]

4 Clinical Use

Type of cytotoxic: Antimetabolite.

Main indications: Palliative treatment of a variety of carcinomas both alone and in combination.

Dosage: Up to 15 mg/kg IV once weekly, maximum daily dose 1 g. Fluorouracil may be used as an induction once daily for five to seven days or in a three to four week cycle as part of combination therapy. Also, 5 to 7.5 mg/kg by continuous intra-arterial infusion over 24 hours has been used.

5 Preparation of Injection

Dilution: May be administered undiluted or diluted as an infusion.

Bolus administration: Administer injection slowly directly into the vein or via a fast-running drip.

Infusion: Diluted in 5% glucose or 0.9% sodium chloride and administered over four to 24 hours.

Gloves for handling: Rubber or PVC should be used.

Extravasation: Non-irritant. No special treatment required.

6 Destruction of Drug or Contaminated Articles

Incineration: 700°C.

Chemical: 5% sodium hypochlorite/24 hours.

Contact with skin: Wash thoroughly with soap and water.

References

1. Quebbeman, E.J. *et al.* (1984). Stability of fluorouracil in plastic containers used for continuous infusion at home. *Am. J. Hosp. Pharm.* **41**, 1153–1156.
2. Vincke, A.E. *et al.* (1989). Extended stability of 5-fluorouracil and methotrexate solutions in PVC containers. *Int. J. Pharm.* **54**, 181–189.
3. Allen, V.J. *et al.* (1988). Stability study of fluorouracil administered using a constant infusion pump. American Society of Hospital Pharmacists Meeting, **23**, 387.
4. Sesin, G.P. *et al.* (1982). Stability study of 5-fluorouracil following repackaging in plastic disposable syringes and multidose vials. *Am. J. Intraven. Ther. Clin. Nutrition,* **9**, 23–25, 29–30.
5. Sewell, G.J. (1988). *Cancer chemotherapy by infusion: drug stability and compatibility considerations.* Proc. Int. Symposium on Oncological Pharmacy Practice, Rotorua, New Zealand, 253–278.
6. Personal communication, David Bull Laboratories. (1985). Data on file.
7. Benvenuto, J.A. *et al.* (1981). Stability and compatibility of antitumour agents in glass and plastic containers. *Am. J. Hosp. Pharm.* **38**, 1914–1918.
8. Dorr, R.T. *et al.* (1982). Bleomycin compatibility with selected intravenous medications. *J. Medicine,* **13**, 121–130.
9. McRae, M.P. and King, J.C. (1976). Compatibility of antineoplastic, antibiotic and corticosteroid drugs in intravenous admixtures. *Am. J. Hosp. Pharm.* **33**, 1010–1013.
10. Leonard, S.L. *et al.* (1988). Stability of 5-fluorouracil and leucovorin calcium combined in a single infusion for intravenous administration. American Society of Hospital Pharmacists Mid-year Clinical Meeting **23**, 48.
11. Lokich, J. *et al.* (1989). Cyclophosphamide, methotrexate and 5-fluorouracil in a three-drug admixture. *Cancer,* **63**, 822–824.
12. Dorr, R.T. (1979). Incompatibilities with parenteral and anticancer drugs. *Am. J. Intraven. Ther. Clin. Nutrition* **6**, 42,45,46,52.

Prepared by R.J. Needle

IDARUBICIN

1 General Details

Approved name: Idarubicin.

Proprietary name: Zavedos.

Manufacturer or supplier: Farmitalia Carlo Erba Ltd.

Presentation and formulation details: Sterile, pyrogen-free, orange-red, freeze-dried powder in vials containing 5 mg and 10 mg of idarubicin hydrochloride, with 50 mg and 100 mg of lactose respectively. There are no preservatives in the preparation.[1] Capsules (5 mg and 10 mg) are also available on a named patient basis.[2]

Storage and shelf-life of unopened container: Dry, unopened vials expire three years from the date of manufacture when stored in a dry place protected from sunlight. Vials of idarubicin are stored at room temperature.[2]

2 Chemistry

Type: A cytotoxic antibiotic consisting of an aminosugar daunosamine, linked through a glycosidic bond to the C7 of a tetracyclic aglycone, 4-demethoxydaunorubicinone.

Molecular structure:

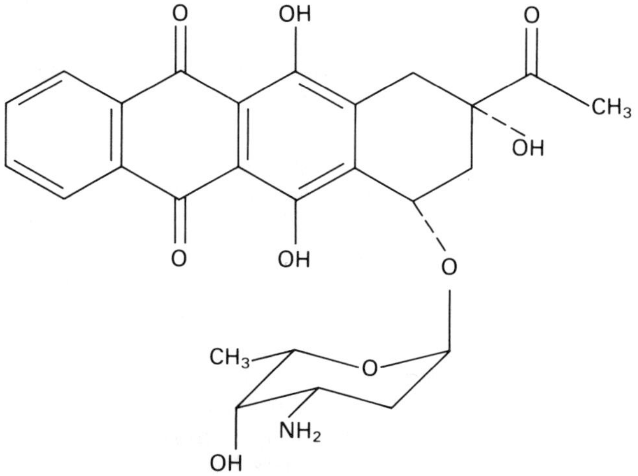

Molecular weight: 533.97.

Solubility: Idarubicin is sparingly soluble in water for injections, 5% glucose, 0.9% sodium chloride, slightly soluble in ethanol and practically insoluble in non-polar organic solvents.[3]

3 Stability Profile

Physical and chemical stability: The manufacturer states that the reconstituted solution is chemically stable for at least 48 hours at 2 to 8°C and 24 hours at room temperature.[1] Very few data on the long-term stability of idarubicin are available.

The stability of the anthracyclines, as a group, is dependent on a number of factors, including the pH of the medium. They are also light sensitive and adsorb on to glass and certain plastics.

Effect of pH: The rate of cleavage of the glycosidic bond in acidic media is strongly dependent on structural modifications in the amino sugar moiety and unaffected by structural modifications in the aglycone portion of the molecule.[4] As daunorubicin and idarubicin both possess daunosamine as the sugar moiety, the rate of degradation of these three analogues is expected to be similar in acidic solution. There are no published data available to confirm this hypothesis.

Acidic hydrolysis of idarubicin, shown in Figure 1, is expected to yield a red-coloured, water-insoluble aglycone, 4-demethoxy-daunorubicinone, and a water-soluble amino sugar, daunosamine.

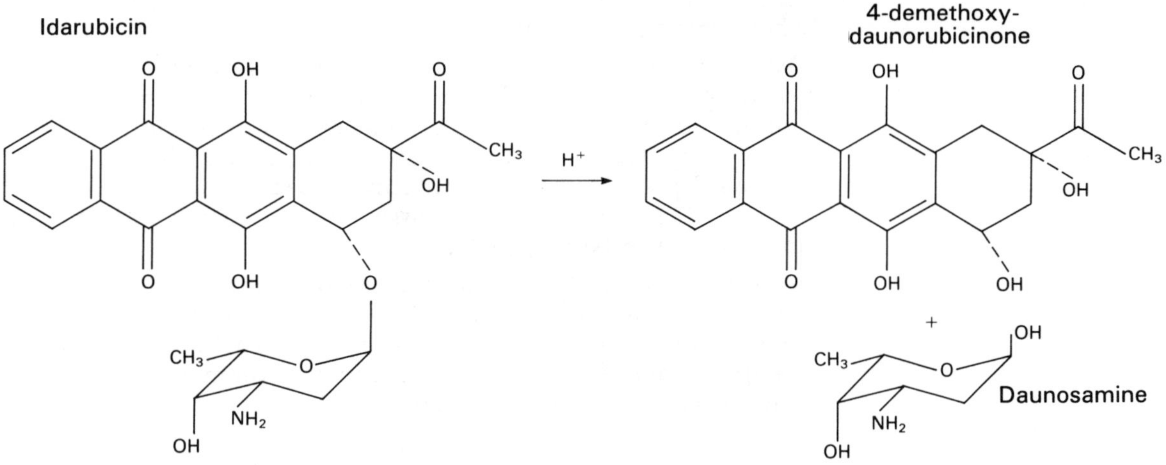

Figure 1: *Proposed degradation pathway for idarubicin in acidic solution*

There are no data available on the degradation of idarubicin in alkaline solution. The manufacturers recommend that prolonged contact of idarubicin with any solution of alkaline pH should be avoided as it will result in degradation.[1]

In alkaline solution, the rate of degradation of the anthracyclines is affected by structural modifications in the aglycone portion of the molecule and unaffected by structural modifications in the amino sugar moiety.[4] As idarubicin possesses a unique aglycone, 4-demethoxydaunorubicinone, its stability in alkaline media cannot be predicted from existing data for the other anthracyclines. For this reason, it is imperative that more stability studies are undertaken with this analogue.

Effect of light: Data on the photodegradation of doxorubicin have been published[5] but there are no data available for idarubicin. The rates of photodegradation of doxorubicin, daunorubicin and epirubicin have been reported to be similar and may be substantial at concentrations below 100 µg/ml if solutions are exposed to light for sufficient time.[6] At higher concentrations, such as those used for cancer chemotherapy (at least 500 µg/ml), no special precautions are necessary to protect freshly prepared solutions of doxorubicin, daunorubicin and epirubicin from light.[6] The manufacturers suggest that idarubicin is treated in a similar fashion to these other anthracyclines and that no precautions are necessary to protect freshly prepared solutions of idarubicin from light.[2]

Effect of temperature: A review of the literature reveals one well-controlled study in which idarubicin was observed to be stable in polypropylene tubes, in 5% glucose (pH 4.7), 3.3% glucose with 0.3% sodium chloride (pH 4.4), lactated Ringer's solution (pH 6.8) and 0.9% sodium chloride (pH 7.0) for 28 days when stored in the dark at 25°C.[7]

Container compatibility: Idarubicin is compatible with polypropylene, PVC and glass.[2] Doxorubicin, daunorubicin and epirubicin adsorb onto glass but not on to siliconized glass or polypropylene.[8] Idarubicin may behave in a similar manner. In clinical practice, when idarubicin is used at concentrations of at least 500 µg/ml, adsorptive losses during storage and delivery are expected to be negligible.

Compatibility with other drugs: Prolonged contact with any solution of alkaline pH should be avoided as it will result in degradation. Idarubicin should not be mixed with heparin as a precipitate may form. The manufacturer recommends that no other drugs are mixed with idarubicin.[1]

Stability in clinical practice

Idarubicin appears to be chemically stable for at least 28 days in 5% glucose, glucose/saline admixtures and 0.9% sodium chloride at 25°C.[7] After reconstitution, vials of idarubicin should be refrigerated and protected from light.[2]

4 Clinical Use

Main indications: Remission induction in untreated adults with acute non-lymphocytic leukaemia or for remission induction in relapsed or refractory patients. Idarubicin is also indicated in acute lymphocytic leukaemia as second line treatment in adults and children. It may be used in combination regimens with other cytotoxic agents.[1]

Dosage: Dosage is usually calculated on the basis of body surface area. The manufacturer gives the following recommendations for the intravenous preparation:

(a) *Acute non-lymphocytic leukaemia:* In adults the dose schedule suggested is 12 mg/m^2 intravenously daily for three days in combination with cytarabine. Another dosage schedule in which idarubicin has been used as a single agent and in combination is 8 mg/m^2 intravenously daily for five days.

(b) *Acute lymphocytic leukaemia:* As a single agent the suggested dose is 12 mg/m^2 intravenously daily for three days in adults and 10 mg/m^2 intravenously daily for three days in children.

Oral idarubicin has been used in various clinical trials in doses ranging from 20 mg/m^2 to 50 mg/m^2.[2,9]

All of the above dosage schedules should, however, take into account the haematological status of the patient and the dosages of other cytotoxic drugs when used in combination. Idarubicin therapy should not be started in patients with severe renal and liver impairment or patients with uncontrolled infections. In a number of phase III trials, treatment was not given if bilirubin and/or serum creatinine levels exceeded 2 mg/100 ml. With other anthracyclines a 50% dosage reduction is generally employed if bilirubin and creatinine levels are in the range 1.2 to 2.0 mg/100 ml.[1]

On the basis of the recommended dosage schedules the total cumulative dose administered over two courses can be expected to reach 60 to 80 mg/m^2. Although a cumulative dosage limit cannot yet be defined, a specific cardiological evaluation in cancer patients showed no significant modifications of cardiac function in patients treated with idarubicin at a mean cumulative dosage of 95 mg/m^2.[1]

5 Preparation of Injection

Dilution: The contents of the 5 mg vial should be dissolved in 5 ml of water for injections and the 10 mg vial in 10 ml of the same solvent. After addition of the diluent and gentle shaking, the contents of the vial will dissolve to produce a solution of 1 mg/ml.[1]

Bolus administration: Administration is by the intravenous route only. The reconstituted solution should be given over five to ten minutes into the side arm of a freely-running intravenous infusion of 0.9% sodium chloride. This technique minimizes the risk of thrombosis or perivenous extravasation which can lead to severe cellulitis or necrosis.[1]

Infusion: The doses and duration of infusions of idarubicin that have been used in clinical trials range from 8 mg/m^2 to 16 mg/m^2 over four hours, 24 hours or 72 hours.[2,9–11]

Gloves for handling: Rubber gloves are recommended.

Extravasation: Idarubicin is a potent vesicant. Extravasation of idarubicin at the site of injection can cause severe local tissue necrosis. Care should be taken to avoid extravasation by following the recommended procedures for administration. A stinging or burning sensation at the site of administration signifies a degree of extravasation and the infusion should be stopped immediately and resumed in another vein. Appropriate treatment of the extravasated area should be undertaken immediately.[1]

6 Destruction of Drug of Contaminated Articles

Incineration: 700°C.[2]

Chemical: Sodium hypochlorite (1% available chlorine) solution/24 hours.[1]

Contact with skin: Wash with water, or soap and water. If the eyes are contaminated immediate irrigation with 0.9% sodium chloride should be carried out.[1]

References

1. Idarubicin. Data sheet. (1990). Farmitalia Carlo Erba Ltd, St Albans, Herts, UK.
2. Personal communication. Farmitalia Carlo Erba Ltd. Unpublished data.
3. Idarubicin: Summary of preclinical studies up to March 1980. (1990). Cagnasso, M.G. (ed.), Farmitalia Carlo Erba Ltd.
4. Beijnen, J.H. *et al.* (1986). Aspects of the degradation kinetics of doxorubicin in aqueous solution. *Int. J. Pharm.* **32**, 123–131.
5. Tavoloni, N. *et al.* (1980). Photolytic degradation of adriamycin. Communications: *J. Pharm. Pharmacol.* **32**, 860–862.
6. Wood, M.J. *et al.* (1990). Photodegradation of doxorubicin, daunorubicin and epirubicin measured by high-performance liquid chromatography. *J. Clin. Pharm. Ther.* (In Press).
7. Beijnen, J.H. *et al.* (1985). Stability of anthracycline antitumour agents in infusion fluids. *J. Parent. Sci. Technol.* **39**, 220–222.
8. Bosanquet, A.G. (1986). Stability of solutions of antineoplastic agents during preparation and storage for *in vitro* assays. II. Assay methods, Adriamycin and the other antitumour antibiotics. *Cancer Chemother. Pharmacol.* **17**, 1–10.
9. Speth, P.A.J. *et al.* (1986). Plasma and human leukaemic cell pharmacokinetics of oral and intravenous 4-demethoxydaunomycin. *Clin. Pharm. Ther.* **40**, 643–649.
10. Speth, P.A.J. *et al.* (1989). Idarubicin *versus* daunorubicin: Preclinical and clinical pharmacokinetic studies. *Semin. Oncol.* **16**, suppl. 2, 2–9.
11. Vogler, W.R. *et al.* (1988). A phase III trial comparing daunorubicin or idarubicin combined with cytosine arabinoside in acute myelogenous leukaemia (AML). Abstract of two symposia 'XXII Congress of the International Society of Haematology', August 28th–September 2nd, Milan, Italy.

Prepared by M.J. Wood

IFOSFAMIDE

1 General Details

Approved names: Ifosfamide, iphosphamide, isophosphamide.

Proprietary name: Mitoxana.

Manufacturer or supplier: Degussa Pharmaceuticals.

Presentation and formulation details: White freeze-dried powder in glass vials containing 500 mg, 1 g or 2 g ifosfamide. Contains no excipients.

Storage and shelf-life of unopened container: Vials should be stored below 25°C, protected from light;[1] the intact vials are stable for at least five years at 22 to 25°C.[2]

2 Chemistry

Type: Nitrogen mustard.

Molecular structure: N,3-(2-chloroethyl)tetrahydro-2H-1,2,3 Oxaphosphorin-2-amine.

$$\text{NHCH}_2\text{CH}_2\text{Cl}$$
$$\text{CH}_2\text{CH}_2\text{Cl}$$

Molecular weight: 261.1.

Solubility: In water: 1 in 10; in methylene chloride up to 1 g/ml and in carbon disulphide 15 mg/ml. Readily soluble in ethanol.

3 Stability Profile

Physical and chemical stability

Ifosfamide is relatively stable after reconstitution.

Effect of pH: No information available.

Effect of light: Infusions should be protected from light during storage. Light protection during administration is not necessary. Reconstitution of ifosfamide with water for injections containing benzyl alcohol (0.9%) resulted in the formation of two separate liquid phases.[6] Ifosfamide should, therefore, be reconstituted with unpreserved water for injections.

Container compatibility: Compatible with glass, PVC and polypropylene[3] containers.

Compatibility with other drugs: Compatible with mesna (*see* mesna monograph for details).

Stability in clinical practice

Reconstituted solutions are chemically stable for seven days at room temperature and for six weeks under refrigeration.[2,3] Ifosfamide infusion 50 mg/ml in 10 ml polypropylene syringes showed no drug loss over seven days at 4 and 20°C. Combinations of ifosfamide (50 mg/ml) and mesna (40 mg/ml) in 10 ml syringes were stable for 28 days at 4 and 20°C.[4] Ifosfamide (50 mg/ml) and combinations of ifosfamide with mesna (each 50 mg/ml) showed no drug loss at 37°C over 24 hours.[5]

Dilutions of the reconstituted solution to 16 and 0.6 mg/ml concentrations in the following intravenous infusion solutions results in 1 to 5% decomposition in seven days at room temperature and no decomposition in six weeks under refrigeration:[2]

Glucose 5% in Ringer's Injection, lactated
Glucose 5% in sodium chloride 0.9%
Glucose in water
Ringer's Injection, lactated
Sodium chloride 0.45%
Sodium chloride 0.9%
Sodium lactate 1/6 M

4 Clinical Use

Type of cytotoxic agent: Alkylating agent of the nitrogen-mustard type, activated by hepatic microsomal enzymes to produce anti-tumour metabolites.

Main indications: Tumours of the lung, ovary, cervix, breast and testis and soft-tissue sarcoma. Ifosfamide also produces response in osteosarcoma, malignant lymphoma, carcinoma of the pancreas, head and neck tumours and acute leukaemias (except AML).

Dosage: Ifosfamide should not be used without the concurrent administration of mesna (*see* mesna monograph).

The usual dose for each course is 8 to 10 g/m^2, equally fractionated as single daily doses over five days or alternatively, 5 to 6 g/m^2 (maximum of 10 g) administered as a 24-hour infusion. Courses are normally repeated at intervals of two to four weeks for intermittent therapy or three to four weeks for 24-hour infusions. The white cell count should not be less than 4×10^3/mm^3 and the platelet count not less than 100×10^3/mm^3 before starting each course. Usually, four courses are given but up to seven (six by 24 hour infusion) have been administered.

5 Preparation of Injection

Reconstitution: The injection should be reconstituted to give a solution of approximately 8% (80 mg/ml) using:

▼ 6.5 ml water for injections with 500 mg ifosfamide
▼ 12.5 ml water for injections with 1 g ifosfamide
▼ 25 ml water for injections with 2 g ifosfamide

The 8% solution may be:

▼ Diluted to less than 4% and injected into the vein with the patient supine.
▼ Infused in 5% glucose-saline or normal saline over 30 to 120 minutes.

▼ Injected directly into a fast-running infusion, or
▼ Made up in 3 × 1 l glucose-saline or normal saline (each bag made freshly before administration and run in over eight hours).

Bolus administration: May be infused in 5% glucose, glucose-saline or 0.9% sodium chloride infusion over 30 to 120 minutes, or infused over 24 hours in 3 × 1 l glucose-saline or normal saline infusions. (*See* also section on Preparation of Injection.)

Gloves for handling: Rubber gloves of surgical thickness are recommended.

Extravasation: Non-irritant. No specific measures need to be taken and local tissue damage is unlikely.

6 Destruction of Drug or Contaminated Waste

Incineration: 1000°C.

Chemical: 2 N sodium hydroxide in dimethyl formamide/ 24 hours.

Contact with skin: Wash with water.

7 References

1. ABPI Data Sheet Compendium 1989/90. (1989). Datapharm Publications Ltd, London, pp. 216–218.
2. Trissell, L.A. *et al.* (1979). Investigational drug information: ifosfamide and semustine. *Drug Intell. Clin. Pharm.* **13**, 340–343.
3. Trissel, L.A. *et al.* (1985). *Investigational drugs pharmaceutical data*, NCI. Bethesda, Maryland, USA.
4. Adams, P.S. *et al.* (1987). Pharmaceutical aspects of home infusion therapy for cancer patients. *Pharm, J.* **238**, 476–478.
5. Sewell, G.J. and Palmer, A. (1987). Internal report of Exeter Health Authority. *Cytotoxic drugs – stability under in-use conditions.*
6. Behme, R.J. *et al.* (1988). Incompatibility of ifosfamide with benzyl-alcohol-preserved bacteriostatic water for injections. *Am. J. Hosp. Pharm.* **45**, 627–628.

Prepared by G.J. Sewell

MELPHALAN

1 General Details

Approved names: Melphalan, phenylalanine mustard, L-sarcolysine.

Proprietary name: Alkeran.

Manufacturer or supplier: Calmic Medical Division, The Wellcome Foundation Ltd.

Presentation and formulation details: 100 mg sterile anhydrous melphalan in 20 ml vial with an ampoule of solvent containing 1.8 ml of 0.086 ml hydrochloric acid in 36% ethanol and an ampoule of sterile diluent containing 108 mg dipotassium phosphate, 6 ml propylene glycol and water for injections to 9 ml.

Storage and shelf-life of unopened container: The shelf-life is three years when stored between 15 and 25°C and protected from light.

2 Chemistry

Type: Alkylating agent related to nitrogen mustard.

Molecular structure: 4-[bis(2-chloroethyl)amino]-L-phenylalanine.

COOH
|
NH$_2$ — C — H
|
CH$_2$
|
(benzene ring)
|
N(CH$_2$CH$_2$Cl)$_2$

Molecular weight: 305.2 (base); 345.9 (hydrochloride).

Solubility: Practically insoluble in water, soluble in ethanol.

3 Stability Profile

Physical and chemical stability

The reconstituted drug is relatively unstable. The rate of degradation is influenced by temperature, aqueous vehicle and pH.[1] The degradation products are also less water-soluble than melphalan and a precipitate may form on standing, especially in the reconstituted vial.[2] The reconstituted injection retains 90% of its initial potency for approximately 19 hours.

Effect of pH: The drug is most stable at pH 3.0, stability is slightly reduced at pH 5 to 7 but substantially reduced at pH 9.0. Data from Tali and Cradock (1984)[2] have quantified this effect:

pH (buffer)	$T^{1/2}$
3.0	5.3h
5.0	4.9h
7.0	4.8h
9.0	3.9h

The addition of reconstituted injection to infusions will tend to acidify such solutions. The pH of infusions after adding melphalan injection (final concentration 40 µg/ml) are as follows:[1]

infusion fluid	pH
5% glucose	4.1
0.9% sodium chloride	4.2
Ringer's lactate	5.9

Effect of chloride ions: Studies have shown that chloride reduces the rate of hydrolysis of melphalan.[1,4] For example, $t_{90\%}$ of melphalan in 5% glucose is 1.5 hours and in 0.9% sodium chloride is 4.5 hours at 20°C.

Studies[1] provide some evidence of the significance of storage temperature on rates of degradation. Increasing the temperature from 15 to 20°C raised the degradation rate by approximately 25% in various infusion fluids. Unfortunately no studies were conducted under refrigerated storage, but the manufacturer suggests the drug may precipitate on refrigeration.

Effect of light: No information available.

Degradation pathways: Melphalan is degraded to mono-hydroxy-melphalan (II), and then to di-hydroxy-melphalan (III).[2] The kinetics can be described as pseudo-first order (*see* Figure 1).[1,4]

Degradation products are said to be much less cytotoxic.[6]

Container compatibility: Melphalan is compatible with plastic containers, administration sets and plastic syringes.[6]

Compatibility with other drugs: No information available.

Stability in clinical practice

Reconstituted vials must be used or further diluted within 15 to 30 minutes. They can be further diluted on 0.9% sodium chloride and infused over two hours. The diluted drug should not be stored for longer than two hours at ambient temperature (refrigeration may cause precipitation). Melphalan is not absorbed by in-line filters.[5] It is also suggested that solutions of melphalan can be stored frozen in 0.9% sodium chloride for six months without undergoing significant degradation.[5]

No special precautions are required to protect the injection from normal lighting conditions; however, exposure to strong daylight should be avoided.

4 Clinical Use

Type of cytotoxic: Alkylating agent.

Main indications: Localized malignant melanomas; localized soft tissue sarcoma of the extremities.

Dosage: 1 mg/kg administered intravenously, or intra-arterial perfusion of 70 to 100 mg through the part of the body affected by the tumour.

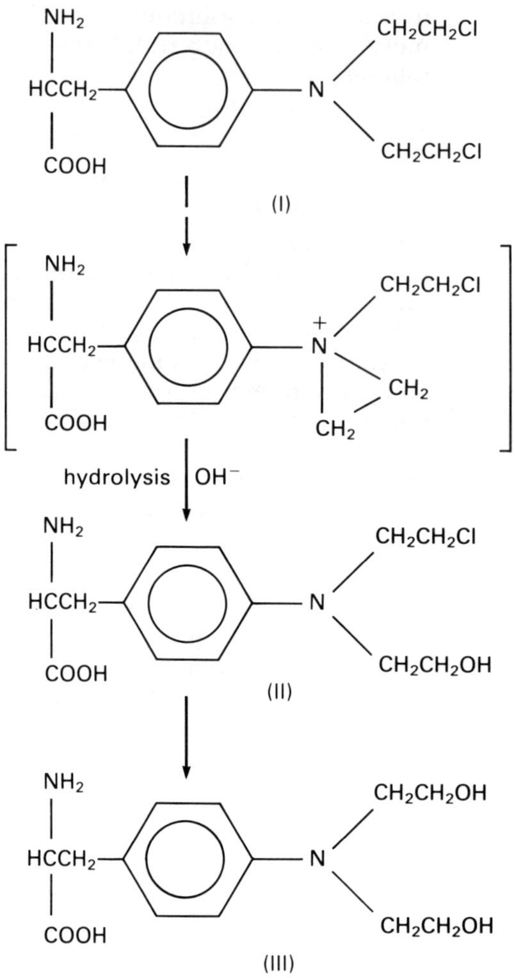

Figure 1. *Degradation of melphalan, 1st-step hydrolysis*

5 Preparation of Injection

Reconstitution: Add 1.8 ml acid-alcohol solvent to the vial containing 100 mg melphalan. Shake to dissolve (about two minutes), then add 9 ml diluent and shake.

Bolus administration: Inject within 15 to 30 minutes of preparation into the tubing of a fast-running infusion.

Infusion of local tissue by perfusion: Dilute in up to 500 ml of 0.9% sodium chloride to give a solution containing 0.4 mg/ml, and infuse slowly for up to two hours. Consult relevant literature for details and alternative methods of tissue perfusion.

Gloves for handling: PVC gloves are recommended.

Extravasation: Not very irritant; treat symptomatically.

6 Destruction of Drug or Contaminated Articles

Incineration: 500°C.

Chemical: 5% sodium thiosulphate in sodium hydroxide solution/24 hours.

Contact with skin: Wash with water.

References

1. Flora, K.P. *et al.* (1979). Application of a simple HPLC method for the determination of melphalan in the presence of its hydrolysis products. *J. Chromatogr.* **177**, 91–97.
2. Tali, S.E. and Cradock, J.C. (1984). Stability of melphalan in infusion fluids. *Am. J. Hosp. Pharm.* **41**, 1380–1382.
3. Trissel, L.A. (1988). *Handbook of injectable drugs*, 5th edn. American Society of Hospital Pharmacists, Bethesda, Maryland, USA.
4. Chang, S.Y. *et al.* (1978). Hydrolysis and protein binding of melphalan. *J. Pharm. Sci.* **67**, 682–684.
5. Bosanquet, A.G. (1985). Stability of solutions of melphalan during preparation and storage for *in vitro* chemosensitivity assays. *J. Pharm. Sci.* **74**, 348–351.
6. Unpublished data, Calmic Medical Division.

Prepared by M.C. Allwood

MESNA

1 General Details

Approved name: Mesna.

Proprietary name: Uromitexan.

Manufacturer or supplier: Degussa Pharmaceuticals.

Presentation and formulation details: Clear glass ampoules containing an aqueous solution of mesna, 400 mg in 4 ml and 1000 mg in 10 ml.

Each ampoule contains:

Mesna	100 mg/ml
Disodium edetate	0.25 mg/ml
Sodium hydroxide as buffer	(q.s.)

Storage and shelf-life of unopened container: When stored below 30°C and protected from light, mensa has a shelf-life of five years.[1]

2 Chemistry

Type: Sulphydryl compound (not cytotoxic).

Molecular structure: sodium 2-mercapto-ethanesulphonate, $HS-CH_2-CH_2-SO_3.Na$.

Molecular weight: 164.2.

Solubility: Water soluble.

3 Stability Profile

Physical and chemical stability

Mesna degrades by oxidation to form dimers through a disulphide bridge. It is available as an aqueous solution, pH 6.5 to 8.5. Mesna should be protected from light, but it is stable under normal lighting conditions during administration.[2]

Container compatibility: Compatible with glass, PVC and polypropylene.

Compatibility with other drugs: Compatible with ifosfamide. Compatible with 0.9% sodium chloride, 5% glucose and Ringer's lactate infusions.

Stability in clinical practice

Mesna is stable for up to 24 hours in a solution of 0.9% sodium chloride or in a solution of ifosfamide in 0.9% sodium chloride.[1] Mesna (3.3 g and 5 g/l) and ifosfamide (also at concentrations of 3.3 g and 5 g/l, respectively) were admixed in 5% glucose solution and Ringer's lactate injection. Mesna exhibited about 5% decomposition over 24 hours while ifosfamide showed no decomposition during this period.[2]

Admixtures of mesna (40 mg/ml) and ifosfamide (50 mg/ml) in water for injections (10 ml) were stable in polypropylene syringes at 4 and 20°C over 28 days, with less than 5% loss of each component present.[3] At 50 mg/ml, they were stable for 24 hours at 37°C,[4] thus enabling ambulatory continuous infusion of this regimen.

4 Clinical Use

Type of cytotoxic: Non-cytotoxic, used in the prophylaxis of urothelial toxicity in patients treated with ifosfamide and cyclophosphamide.

Main indications: Cancer chemotherapy in combination with ifosfamide and cyclophosphamide.

Dosage: Where ifosfamide and cyclophosphamide are used as an intravenous bolus injection, mesna is given over 15 minutes at 20% w/w of the oxazaphosphorine and repeated after four and eight hours. The total dose = 60% w/w of oxazaphosphorine dose. This can be increased to 40% w/w given at 0, 3, 6 and 9 hours (total 160% w/w of oxazaphosphorine dose) in children and patients with damaged urothelium.

Where ifosfamide is used as a 24 hour infusion, mesna is used as a concurrent infusion. Initially, 20% (w/w) of the total ifosfamide dose is given as an intravenous bolus injection, then ifosfamide is infused over 24 hours, followed by a further 12 hour infusion of 60% w/w of the ifosfamide dose. This 12 hour infusion can be replaced with bolus injections at 28, 32, 36 hours, each of 20% of ifosfamide dose, or by oral mesna.

Oral mesna can be used with intermittent oxazaphosphorine therapy or following 24 hour infusion.

The first dose of 40% w/w of mensa is given with the oxazaphosphorine or as the infusion is stopped and repeated at four and eight hours.

5 Preparation of Injection

Dilution: Use undiluted for bolus administration. Add to oxazaphosphorine infusion for 24 hour infusion regimens.
For oral administration, mesna should be taken in a soft drink immediately after opening the ampoule.

Bolus administration: Mesna is given over 15 minutes as 20% of the oxazaphosphorine dose and is repeated after four and eight hours.

Infusion administration: Mesna is given as a concurrent infusion. Initially 20% of the oxazaphosphorine dose is given by intravenous bolus injection, followed by the oxazaphosphorine dose over 24 hours. A further infusion of 60% w/w of the oxazaphosphorine dose is then given.

Gloves for handling: Mesna is not cytotoxic or irritant.

Extravasation: Mesna is not cytotoxic.

6 Destruction of Drug or Contaminated Articles

Mesna is not cytotoxic.

References

1. ABPI Data Sheet Compendium 1989/90. (1989). Datapharm Publications Ltd, London, pp. 219–220.
2. Trissel, L.A. *et al.* (1985). *Investigational drugs pharmaceutical data.* NCI, Bethesda, Maryland, USA.
3. Adams, P.S. *et al.* (1987). Pharmaceutical aspects of home infusion therapy for cancer patients. *Pharm. J.* **238**, 476–478.
4. Sewell, G.J. and Palmer, A. (1987). Internal report of Exeter Health Authority. *Cytotoxic drugs – stability under in-use conditions.*

Prepared by G.J. Sewell

METHOTREXATE

1 General Details

Approved name: Methotrexate.

Proprietary name: Methotrexate Injection, Methotrexate Powder for Injection, Emtexate, Maxtrex.

Manufacturer or supplier: Lederle Laboratories Ltd, David Bull Laboratories Ltd (DBL), Nordic Pharmaceuticals Ltd, Farmitalia Carlo Erba Ltd.

Presentation and formulation details: All solutions are preservative-free.

Methotrexate (Lederle): Solution for injection: A clear, yellow, sterile, aqueous, isotonic solution containing methotrexate sodium equivalent to 2.5 mg/ml (ampoule), 5 mg/2 ml, 25 mg/ml, 50 mg/2 ml, 100 mg/4 ml, 200 mg/8 ml, 500 mg/20 ml, 1 g/40 ml, 5 g/200 ml of methotrexate per vial, together with sodium chloride and sodium hydroxide to adjust the pH to approximately 8.5. Powder for injection: Vials containing yellow, lyophilized powder of methotrexate sodium, equivalent to 500 mg of methotrexate, which is reconstituted before use with 10 ml of water for injections.

Methotrexate Injection (DBL): A clear, yellow, sterile solution of methotrexate in water for injections with sodium chloride to make the solution isotonic. The pH of the solution is 8.4. It is available in the following strengths and packs: 5 mg/2 ml, 50 mg/2 ml, 100 mg/4 ml, 500 mg/20 ml, 1 g/10 ml.

Emtexate (Nordic): Solution for injection: 5 mg/2 ml (ampoule), 50 mg/2 ml, 250 mg/10 ml, 500 mg/20 ml, 1 g/40 ml, 5 g/200 ml, 1 g/10 ml, 5 g/50 ml single use vials. Freeze-dried powder for injection: 500 mg, 1 g, 5 g single use vials which are reconstituted before use with 10 ml, 20 ml, 48 ml of water for injections respectively.

Maxtrex (Farmitalia Carlo Erba): Vials containing a clear, yellow, sterile solution of methotrexate sodium, 5 mg/2 ml, 50 mg/2 ml, 500 mg/20 ml, 1 g/40 ml, 5 g/200 ml with sodium chloride at pH 8.5.

Storage and shelf-life of unopened containers: All preparations should be stored below 25°C and protected from light.
  The shelf-life is detailed on the package.

2 Chemistry

Type: 4-amino-N-methyl analogue of folic acid.

Molecular structure:

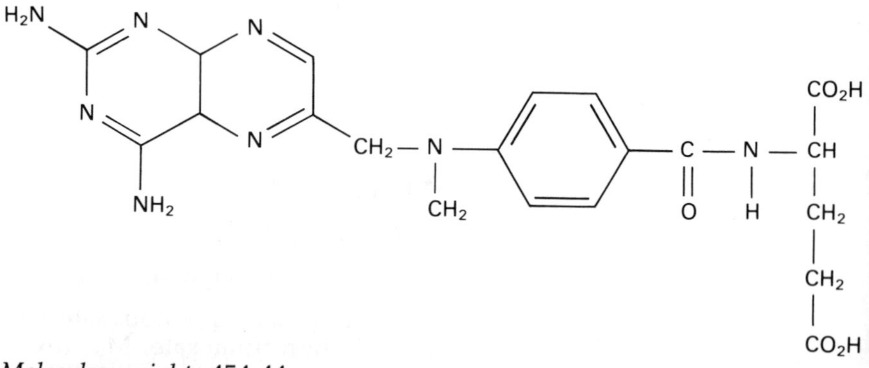

Molecular weight: 454.44.

Solubility: Practically insoluble in water. Very soluble in dilute solutions of alkaline hydroxides and carbonates.[1]

3 Stability Profile

Physical and chemical stability

Methotrexate is relatively stable in aqueous solution provided the recommended storage conditions are observed. The compound is susceptible to both hydrolytic and photolytic degradation. The rate of hydrolytic degradation increases with increase in pH, with minimum degradation occurring between pH 6.6–8.2.[2]

Degradation pathways: The major hydrolytic degradation compound is N-methyl-pteroylglutamic acid (methopterin). The major photolytic degradation compounds are p-aminobenzoylglutamic acid and 2-amino-4-hydroxypteridine-6-carboxylic acid.[3]

Effect of light: The drug is light sensitive and forms a yellow precipitate on prolonged exposure to direct sunlight. Polypropylene and styrene acrylonitrile syringes provided better light protection than did glass ampoules when the drug was stored under controlled light conditions at 25°C. In all cases, no precipitate was observed over a seven-day storage period. Samples stored in the dark showed no evidence of precipitation.[4]

McElnay *et al.*[5] showed that methotrexate 0.1% w/v in 0.9% sodium chloride underwent photodegradation when stored in a range of burette administration sets (Avon Medical) for up to 48 hours. The photodegradation occurred more rapidly in the presence of direct sunlight. The use of an amber giving set or wrapping a standard set in tin foil largely prevented degradation.

Effect of pH: Methotrexate is a bicarboxylic acid with pKa's in the range 4.8 to 5.5[6] and 2.19 and 4.25.[7] Hence, it is essentially ionized at physiological pH. At pH values between 2.6 and 6.6 the drug is converted to the bicarboxylic acid which is relatively insoluble in aqueous solution and will precipitate. Commercially available injection is stabilized to approximately pH 8.4 with sodium hydroxide. However, dilution in acidic solutions may result in precipitation of the drug.[8] For this reason, dilutions in 5% glucose should be checked carefully for evidence of precipitation.

Container compatibility: At a pH value of 8.4, methotrexate injection is largely ionized and, therefore, is unlikely to exhibit adsorption phenomena. There have been no reports of adsorption of methotrexate to plastic containers.

Although extraction into solution is possible, especially with plastic syringes, the extent and rate of leaching is likely to be low at room temperature.[9,10] It should be noted, however, that 2-mercaptobenzothiazole (a mercaptan present in the rubber plunger) is soluble in alkali and alkali carbonate solutions[7] and may leach into the alkaline methotrexate injection on prolonged storage in plastic syringes. Mercaptans may cause problems as analytical or toxicological contaminants.

Compatibility with other drugs: Methotrexate is chemically and physically incompatible with cytarabine, fluorouracil and prednisolone sodium phosphate.[11] However, another study has shown that admixtures of methotrexate with hydrocortisone sodium succinate and cytarabine in 0.9% sodium chloride injection and 5% glucose injection at two concentrations of the three drugs similar to those of the drugs administered intrathecally were stable for at least 10 hours at 25°C. Thereafter, precipitation was noticed in some of the admixtures.[12]

A recent study[13] investigated the compatibility and stability of cyclophosphamide, methotrexate and 5-fluorouracil in a three-drug admixture. Cyclophosphamide (100 mg), methotrexate (1.5 mg), and 5-fluorouracil (500 mg) were reconstituted in a total volume of 60 ml of normal saline. The solution was maintained at room temperature in PVC plastic reservoir bags (Lifecare 1500 System, Abbott). No significant loss of 5-fluorouracil or methotrexate was observed up to 14 days after reconstitution of the three-drug admixture. However, a 9.3% loss of cyclo-phosphamide was observed, accompanied by the appearance of a degradation product in the HPLC chromatogram after seven days. Control admixtures indicated that the cyclophosphamide and methotrexate were chemically incompatible and that there was a pH change in this admixture from 6.6 to 4.57. At this pH, methotrexate stability is compromised. Based on this information, it may be possible to administer cyclo-phosphamide, methotrexate and 5-fluorouracil as a three-drug admixture in an infusion pump, in the proportions reported, for up to seven days. However, solutions should be checked carefully for precipitation and such admixtures should not be used in implantable infusion pumps.

Methotrexate is partially bound to serum proteins and toxicity may be increased by preparations such as salicylates, diuretics, hypoglycaemics, sulphonamides, diphenylhydantoin, tetracyclines, chloramphenicol and acidic anti-inflammatory agents, by displacement. A number of these drugs will also compete with methotrexate for transport and reduce its renal tubular secretion. In particular, salicylates and sulphonamides should be avoided.[14,15]

Folic acid-containing preparations may alter responses to methotrexate.

Concomitant use of other drugs with nephrotoxic or hepatotoxic potential (including alcohol) should be avoided.

Stability in clinical practice

Although the manufacturers do not recommend re-use of the methotrexate solution, the relative stability of methotrexate in aqueous solution would suggest that, once opened, chemical and physical stability will be preserved, provided the injection is manipulated under aseptic conditions and is stored in the original container at 4 to 8°C in the absence of light. In general, a shelf-life of one month at 4°C after opening would seem to be satisfactory.

Infusions: Information on the stability of the drug, when diluted in the recommended solutions for infusion, is variable. The manufacturers are limited by the terms of their product licences to a maximum shelf-life of 24 hours at 25°C. However, a number of reports suggest that methotrexate is stable over a wide range of concentrations when stored in Viaflex (Baxter Healthcare Ltd) containers for longer than 24 hours.[16–19] In particular, work carried out by Baxter[17] indicated that, at a concentration of 1 to 10 mg/ml in 5% glucose and 1.25 to 12.5 mg/ml in 0.9% sodium chloride infusions, methotrexate was stable for up to one month at 4°C and five days at 25°C when stored in both Baxter infusors and Viaflex minibags.

Further studies[18] on the stability of methotrexate 1.25 to 12.5 mg/ml in 0.9% sodium chloride infusion stored in both glass and PVC containers (Baxter, Viaflex) have shown that the drug is physically and chemically stable for up to 15 weeks at 4°C followed by an additional week of storage at room temperature.

Although there is some evidence that methotrexate infusion solutions prepared in Viaflex minibags can be frozen to −20°C and stored for at least three months without significant reduction in methotrexate concentration or change in pH,[19] the use of microwave ovens to thaw solutions prior to use should not be undertaken without careful validation of the thawing process.

Syringe storage: Methotrexate injection, at a concentration of 50 mg/ml or less, stored in sealed Monoject (Sherwood Medical) or Plastipak (Becton Dickinson) plastic disposable syringes in the absence of light at a temperature not exceeding 25°C is stable (<10% degradation) for a period of up to eight months. Storage in Sabre (Gillette) and Steriseal (NI Ltd) syringes should not exceed 70 days.[4] Experience has shown that for routine use, a shelf-life of one month at 4°C is adequate.

4 Clinical Use

Type of cytotoxic: Antimetabolite.

Main indications: Acute lymphoblastic leukaemia, choriocarcinoma, non-Hodgkin's lymphomas, solid tumours, severe psoriasis.

Dosage and administration: Methotrexate injection may be given by the intramuscular, intravenous, intrathecal, intra-arterial or intraventricular routes. Subcutaneous administration of methotrexate has recently been evaluated.[18] Methotrexate administered by this route is well tolerated and well absorbed.

Dosages vary considerably depending on the condition being treated and are based on the patient's body weight or surface area, except in the case of intrathecal or intraventricular administration when a maximum dose of 15 mg is recommended. See Data Sheet for details of specific regimens.

With high-dose therapy, alkalinization of the urine using sodium bicarbonate 1.2 g orally, four times a day for five days, helps to prevent precipitation of methotrexate in the kidney tubules.

Doses greater than 100 mg should be given by IV infusion over a period not exceeding 24 hours. Lower doses may be given by rapid IV bolus injection over 2 to 3 minutes or by infusion. The concentration of the final injection is not critical.

5 Preparation of Injection

Dilution: The drug may be diluted in 0.9% sodium chloride, 5% glucose, sodium chloride and glucose, compound sodium chloride and compound sodium lactate infusions.

Gloves for handling: Methotrexate is not vesicant and is not likely to be absorbed through intact skin. However, it is an irritant and contact with the skin should be avoided.[8,14,21]

Extravasation: The drug does not cause tissue damage. However, if accidental injection into the tissues occurs, heparin cream may be applied to the affected area.[8]

6 Destruction of Drug or Contaminated Articles

Incineration: 1000°C.[21]

Chemical: None recommended.

Contact with skin: Wash with water and soothe any transient stinging with a bland cream. Irrigate eyes with copious amounts of water or saline. If significant quantities are inhaled or injected, calcium folinate cover should be considered.

References

1. Anon. (1982). *The Extra Pharmacopoeia*, 29th edn. Reynolds, J.E.F. (ed.), The Pharmaceutical Press, London.
2. Hansen, J. *et al.* (1983). Kinetics of degradation of methotrexate in aqueous solution. *Int. J. Pharm.* **16**, 141–152.
3. Chatterji, D.C. and Gallelli, J.F. (1978). Thermal and photolytic decomposition of methotrexate in aqueous solution. *J. Pharm. Sci.* **67**, 526–531.
4. Wright, M.P. and Newton, J.M. (1988). Stability of methotrexate injection in prefilled plastic disposable syringes. *Int. J. Pharm.* **45**, 237–244.
5. McElnay, J.C. *et al.* (1988). Stability of methotrexate and vinblastine in burette administration sets. *Int. J. Pharm.* **47**, 239–247.
6. Bleyer, W.A. (1978). The clinical pharmacology of methotrexate. New applications of an old drug. *Cancer,* **41**, 36–50.
7. The Merck Index, 10th edn. (1983). Merck and Co. Inc., Rathway, New Jersey, USA.
8. Nordic Pharmaceuticals Ltd. (1985). Personal communication.
9. Sherwood Medical Ltd. (1984). Personal communication.
10. Gillette UK Ltd. (1984). Personal communication.

11. D'Arcy, P.F. (1983). Reactions and interactions in handling anticancer drugs. *Drug Intell. Clin. Pharm.* **17**, 532–538.
12. Cheung, Y. *et al.* (1984). Stability of cytarabine, methotrexate sodium and hydrocortisone sodium succinate admixtures. *Am. J. Hosp. Pharm.* **41**, 1802–1806.
13. Lokich, J. *et al.* (1989). Cyclophosphamide, methotrexate, and 5-fluorouracil in a three-drug admixture. Phase 1 trial of 14-day continuous ambulatory infusion. *Cancer,* **63**, 822–824.
14. ABPI Data Sheet Compendium 1989/90. (1989). Datapharm Publications Ltd, London, pp. 470–471, 766–769.
15. Balis, F.M. *et al.* (1983). Clinical pharmacokinetics of commonly used anticancer drugs. *Clin. Pharmacokinet.* **8**, 202–232.
16. Roach, M. (1979). Methotrexate infusions, *Pharm. J.* **223**(6050), 557.
17. Baxter Healthcare Ltd. (1985). Information chart.
18. Vincke, B.J. *et al.* (1989). Extended stability of 5-fluorouacil and methotrexate solutions in PVC containers. *Int. J. Pharm.* **54**, 181–189.
19. Dyvik, O. *et al.* (1986). Methotrexate in infusion solutions – a stability test for the hospital pharmacy. *J. Clin. Hosp. Pharm.* **11**, 343–348.
20. Balis, F.M. *et al.* (1988). Pharmacokinetics of subcutaneous methotrexate. *J. Clin. Oncol.* **6**, 1882–1886.
21. Bristol-Myers Pharmaceuticals. (1985). Personal communication.

Prepared by M.P. Wright

MITHRAMYCIN

1 General Details

Approved names: Mithramycin, plicamycin.

Proprietary name: Mithracin.

Manufacturer or supplier: Pfizer Ltd.

Presentation and formulation details: Yellow lyophilized powder in vial, containing 2.5 mg mithramycin. Contains 100 mg mannitol and disodium hydrogen phosphate to adjust pH to 7.0 after reconstitution.

Storage and shelf-life of unopened container: Shelf-life of two years when stored in a refrigerator at 2 to 8°C and protected from light; shelf-life of six months at room temperature.

2 Chemistry

Type: Cytotoxic antibiotic.

Molecular structure: (See p. 189.)

Solubility: Soluble in water.

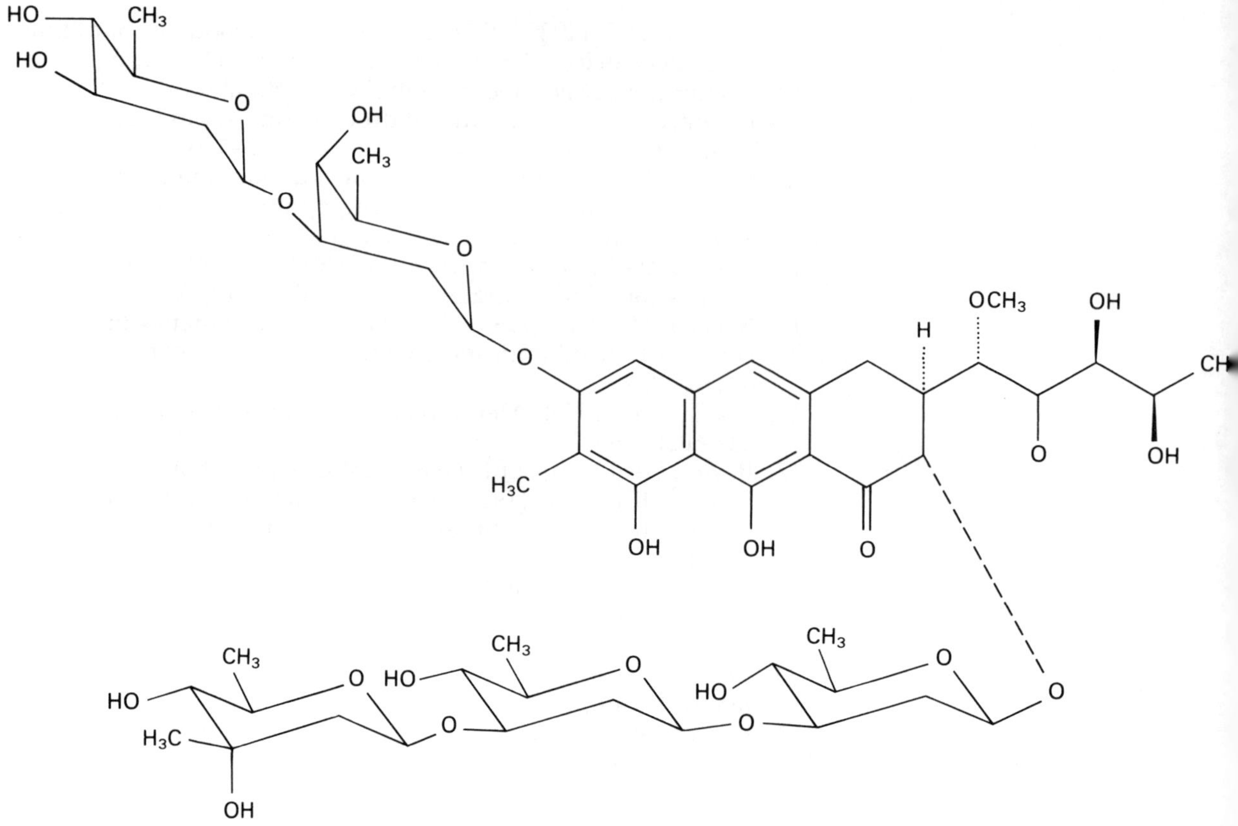

Molecular weight: 1085.2.

3 Stability Profile

Physical and chemical stability

The dry powder is stable for six months at ambient temperature.[1] The drug in aqueous solution decomposes in acid or alkaline conditions. The pH of an aqueous solution (0.5 mg/ml) is 4.5 to 5.5, although the injection is buffered to pH 7. Losses of about 13% at pH 4 to 5 and ambient temperature after 24 hours have been reported.[2] Solutions at pH 5 to 7.5 are stable for at least two days at 2 to 6°C.

Effect of light: The drug is described as relatively sensitive to light, and direct exposure to strong daylight should be avoided.

Degradation pathways: Acid hydrolysis (below pH 5.0) yields a number of degradation products, including chromomycinone D, mycarose, D olivose and D oliose.[2] The relative toxicity of these compounds is unknown.

Compatibility information: Mithramycin will chellate metals, such as iron.

Compatibility with containers: Compatible with PVC.[2]

Stability in clinical practice

The drug is relatively stable after reconstitution with water for injections and may be stored for two days at 2 to 6°C. The drug may be further diluted in 5% glucose (other infusion fluids are not recommended), although some degradation may occur indicating storage is undesirable. Such dilutions are quite stable (less than 10% loss) for 24 hours at room temperature in either glass or PVC containers, or 48 hours at 2 to 6°C.[2] However, the presence of degradation productions is undesirable, so it is recommended the diluted injection be used immediately. It is reported that mithramycin binds to cellulose acetate in-line filters, approximately 14% of the dose being removed during passage of a solution in 5% glucose through an in-line filter.[4]

4 Clinical Use

Type of cytotoxic: Anti-tumour antibiotic.

Main indications: Refractory hypercalcaemia.

Dosage: 25 µg/kg/day for three to four day periods.

5 Preparation of Injection

Dilution: Add 4.9 ml water for injections and shake to dissolve. The solution contains 500 µg/ml. It may be stored for short periods at 2 to 6°C, but this is not recommended by the manufacturer.

Bolus administration: Not recommended.

Intravenous infusion: The required volume of the reconstituted injection is added to 1 l of 5% glucose. Inject slowly over four to six hours (200 ml/h). The infusion may be stored at 2 to 6°C for up to 24 hours.

Gloves for handling: PVC gloves with rubber over-gloves are recommended.

Extravasation: Moderately damaging. There is no known antidote.

Application of moderate heat to the site of extravasation is recommended to disperse the drug and reduce discomfort.

6 Destruction of Drug or Contaminated Article

Incineration: 1000°C.

Chemical: 10% w/v trisodium phosphate (or 0.1 M sodium hydroxide).

Contact with skin: Wash affected area with copious amounts of water.

References

1. Wolfert, R.R. and Cox, R.M. (1975). Room temperature stability of drug products labelled for refrigeration storage. *Am. J. Hosp. Pharm.* **32**, 585–587.
2. Cheng, C.C. and Kwang-Yeun, Z. (1972). Some antineoplastic antibiotics. *J. Pharm. Sci.* **61**, 4.

3. Bosanquet, A.G. (1986). Stability of solutions of anti-neoplastic agents during preparation and storage for *in vitro* assays. II. Assay methods, Adriamycin and the other anti-tumour antibiotics. *Cancer Chemother. Pharmacol.* **17**, 1–10.
4. Butler, L.D. *et al.* (1980). Effect of in-line filtration on the potency of low-dose drugs. *Am. J. Hosp. Pharm.* **37**, 935–941.

Prepared by M.C. Allwood

MITOMYCIN

1 General Details

Approved names: Mitomycin C, Mitomycin X.

Proprietary name: Mitomycin C Kyowa.

Manufacturer or supplier: Martindale Pharmaceuticals Ltd.

Presentation and formulation details: Purple powder in vials containing 2 mg, 10 mg or 20 mg mitomycin C. The 2 mg vial contains 48 mg sodium chloride and the 10 mg vial contains 240 mg sodium chloride.

   The diluent for the USP formulation is mannitol (Mutamycin, Bristol Laboratories Ltd).

Storage and shelf-life of unopened container: Four years at ambient temperature and protected from light.

2 Chemistry

Molecular Structure: 1 S-(1,8,8a,8b) -6-amino-8- (amino-carbonyl)oxy methyl -1,1,2,8,8a,8b-hexahydro-methoxy-5-methyl-azirino 2′,3′,4,7, pyrrolo 1,2- indole-4,7-dione.

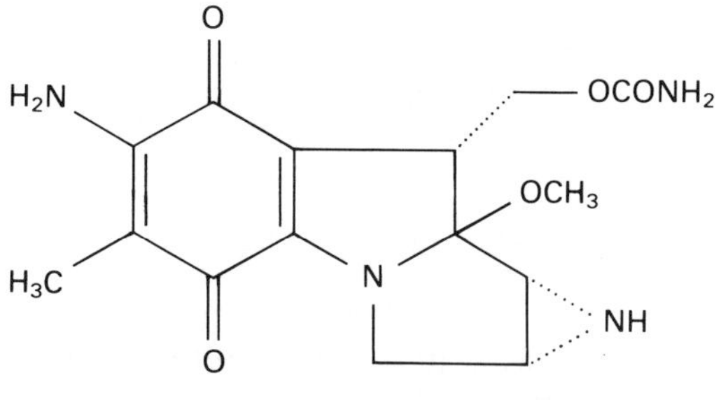

O
H₂N — OCONH₂
OCH₃
N
H₃C
NH
O

Molecular weight: 349.
Solubility: Sparingly soluble in water.

3 Stability Profile

Physical and chemical stability

Relatively unstable in aqueous solution, losing about 20% potency at room temperature in three days, according to the UK supplier. It should be noted that early studies[1] suggested that the reconstituted drug was stable for 72 hours at 2 to 6°C in water for injections. This information was not supported by adequate data. Stability is pH-dependent and is greatest between pH 7 and 8. Mitomycin is significantly less stable in acid conditions. One report has indicated a degradation rate constant of 5×10^{-6} s^{-1} at pH 4.9 and 20°C.[2]

Degradation pathways: See[2] for a recent summary.

In alkali the 7 amino group is replaced by an hydroxyl group while the remainder of the mitosane skeleton remains intact.

In acid the methoxy group is cleaved to form a 9-9a unsaturated bond. Also the 1,2 – fused aziridine ring is opened to give 2 isomeric compounds 1 and 2, with an hydroxyl group at position 1 and amino group at position 2:

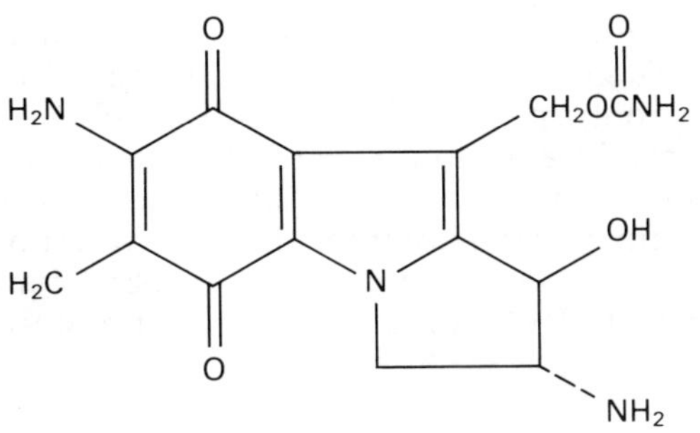

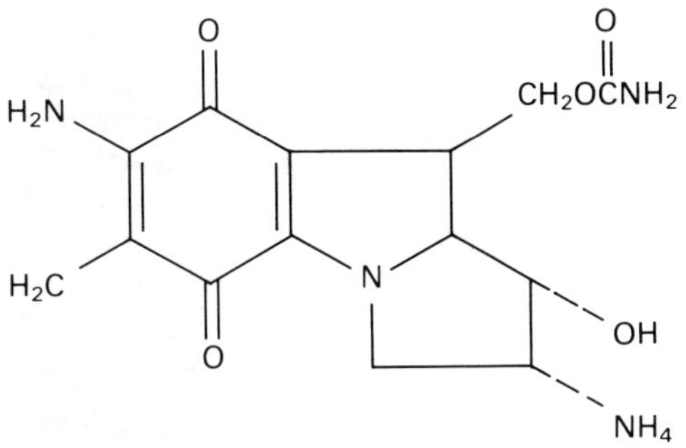

Degradation rate is related to temperature after reconstitution. The reconstituted drug is significantly more stable at 2 to 6°C compared to ambient conditions. However, solubility is reduced substantially in the refrigerator and solutions containing 0.5 mg/ml in water for injections may precipitate at 2 to 6°C. The reconstituted drug should be protected from daylight, although light-induced degradation would not normally be a significant factor during bolus administration.

Container compatibility: There is no information to indicate that stability or compatibility are affected by storage in plastic syringes.

Infusion containers: Studies suggest that stability is not greatly influenced by the nature of the container in which the drug is diluted (glass bottles, PVC containers, Viaflex), when the dilution vehicle is 0.9% sodium chloride infusion.[3]

Administration sets: No information available. However, the studies would suggest that mitomycin does not adsorb significantly to standard administration sets.[3]

Compatibility with other drugs: Mitomycin may be mixed with bleomycin if used immediately but depends on concentration.[4] Some degradation of bleomycin was reported, mitomycin stability was not assessed. Trissel[1] indicates that heparin is compatible.

Stability in clinical practice

Current guidelines from the UK supplier recommend that reconstituted vials are stable for 12 hours if stored at room temperature. Refrigeration may cause precipitation and is not, therefore, recommended. The drug may be further diluted, preferably in 0.9% sodium chloride. In 5% glucose, the diluted infusion should be used immediately, whilst it may be stored for not more than 12 hours in 0.9% sodium chloride. Few studies have been reported on stability after dilution in infusion fluids. One report[3] indicates that degradation is more rapid in 5% glucose than in 0.9% sodium chloride. The studies suggest an initial rapid fall (about 10 to 15%) in content after dilution. However, these studies have not been repeated and remain controversial.

The stability of mitomycin was also studied in 0.9% sodium chloride and 5% glucose, with or without buffering, stored in PVC containers.[5] The drug, at a concentration of 50 µg/ml, was unstable in both (unbuffered) vehicles. There was about 75% degradation in 5% glucose after 12 hours storage at room temperature. In contrast, if vehicles were phosphate-buffered to pH 7.8, mitomycin appeared to be stable for more than 120 days at 5°C. These results, however, have been questioned.[6] In a further study, unbuffered solutions in 0.9% sodium chloride were reported to be stable when stored at −30°C for at least 28 days.[7] Sorption to PVC containers does not appear to occur.[8]

4 Clinical Use

Type of cytotoxic: Anti-tumour antibiotic.

Main indications: Bladder, rectal and skin cancer.

Dosage: 4 to 10 mg (0.06–0.15 mg/kg) at one to six weekly intervals; up to 40 to 80 mg (2 mg/kg) cumulative doses have been given in some treatments.

5 Preparation of Injection

Reconstitution: solutions are formed rapidly.

     2 mg vial +   5 ml water for injections = 0.4 mg/ml
    10 mg vial + 10 ml water for injections =   1 mg/ml
    20 mg vial + 20 ml water for injections =   1 mg/ml

May be stored for up to 12 hours at room temperature (do not refrigerate).

Bolus administration: Inject slowly into a vein or slow-running drip at a rate of approximately 1 ml/min or more rapidly into a fast-running drip of 0.9% sodium chloride or 5% glucose. The stability of reconstituted drug in plastic syringes is not known.

Infusion: Dilute with 0.9% sodium chloride (use within 12 hours) or 5% glucose (use immediately) and infuse over one hour.

Gloves for handling: PVC or rubber gloves are recommended.

Extravasation: Very damaging. The antidote is up to 5 ml of 8.4% sodium bicarbonate injection.

6 Destruction of Drug or Contaminated Articles

Incineration: 500°C.

Chemical: 2 to 5% of hydrochloric acid or sodium hydroxide/
12 hours.

Contact with skin: Very irritant, neutralize with several washes of
sodium bicarbonate solution (8.4%) followed by soap and water;
avoid hand creams.

References

1. Trissel, L.A. (1988). *Handbook of injectable drugs*, 5th edn,
   American Society of Hospital Pharmacists, Bethesda,
   Maryland, USA.
2. Beijner, J.H. and Underberg, W.J.M. (1985). Degradation of
   mitomycin C in acidic conditions. *Int. J. Pharm.* **24**, 219–229.
3. Benuvento, J.A. *et al.* (1981). Stability and compatibility
   of antitumour agents in glass and plastic containers.
   Am. J. Hosp. Pharm. **38**, 1914–1918.
4. Dorr, R.T. *et al.* (1982). Bleomycin compatibility with selected
   intravenous medications. *J. Medicine*, **13**, 121–130.
5. Quebberman, E.J. *et al.* (1985). Stability of mitomycin
   admixtures *Am. J. Hosp. Pharm.* **42**, 1750–1754.
6. Keller, J.H. (1986). Stability of mitomycin admixtures.
   Am. J. Hosp. Pharm. **43**, 59–64.
7. Stole, L.M.L. *et al.* (1986). Stability after freezing and
   thawing of solutions of Mitomycin C in plastic minibags for
   intravesical use. *Pharm. Weekbl (Sci. edn.)* **8**, 286–288.
8. Quebberman, E.J. and Hoffman, N.E. (1986) Stability of
   mitomycin admixtures. *Am. J. Hosp. Pharm.* **43**, 64.

Prepared by M.C. Allwood

MITOZANTRONE

1 General Details

Approved name: Mitozantrone.

Proprietary name: Novantrone.

Manufacturer or supplier: Lederle Laboratories Ltd.

Presentation and formulation details: Vials containing mitozantrone
dihydrochloride solution, equivalent to 2 mg/ml mitozantrone.
Solutions of 20 mg in 10 ml, 25 mg in 12.5 ml and 30 mg in
15 ml are available.
Each vial contains:

Mitozantrone (as the dihydrochloride)	– 20 mg, 25 mg or 30 mg
Sodium chloride	– 0.8% (w/v)
Sodium metabisulphite	– 0.01% (w/v)
Sodium acetate	– 0.005% (w/v)
Water for injections	– q.s.

Storage and shelf-life of unopened container: Store at room temperature. Stable for two years from the date of manufacture. Refrigerated storage may cause precipitation which redissolves on warming to room temperature.[1]

2 Chemistry

Type: Anthracenedione.

Molecular structure: 1.4.Dihydroxy-5,8-bis-2-(2-hydroxyethyl) amino ethylamine-9,10-anthraquinone dihydrochloride.

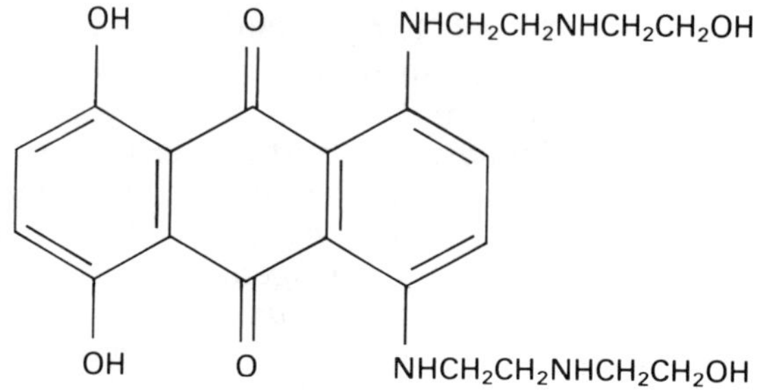

$$\text{OH} \quad \text{O} \quad NHCH_2CH_2NHCH_2CH_2OH$$

$$\text{OH} \quad \text{O} \quad NHCH_2CH_2NHCH_2CH_2OH$$

Molecular weight: 517.4.

Solubility: Water soluble.

3 Stability Profile

Physical and chemical stability

Mitozantrone degrades by oxidation of the phenylenediamine moiety to the corresponding quinoneimine, which then hydrolyses to the quinone.[2]

Effect of pH: Stability is optimal in acidic conditions.

Effect of light: Vials of mitozantrone may precipitate under refrigerated storage. Exposure of vials to sunlight for one month has little effect on the potency and appearance of the product.

Container compatibility: Mitozantrone adsorbs on to glass but not on to polypropylene or PVC.[5]

Compatibility with other drugs: Unstable in alkaline infusions. The injection should not be mixed with infusions containing heparin as precipitation may occur.

Stability in clinical practice

Dilution to 5 mg/l in 0.9% sodium chloride or 5% glucose infusions produced solutions that were physically and chemically compatible, exhibiting no decomposition in 48 hours.[3] The Data Sheet[1] states that dilutions retain potency for 24 hours at room temperature. Polypropylene syringes containing mitozantrone diluted to 2 mg in 10 ml with water for injections (for use in continuous infusion schedules) were found to be stable for 14 days at 4 and 20°C[4] and for 24 hours at 37°C.[5]

4 Clinical Use

Type of cytotoxic: Antibiotic anti-tumour agent.

Indications: Advanced breast cancer, non-Hodgkin's lymphoma, adult acute non-lymphocytic leukaemia in relapse and paediatric leukaemia, hepatoma.

Dosage: As a single agent, 14 mg/m^2 (12 mg/m^2 in patients with low bone marrow reserves).

5. Preparation of Injection

Dilute the required volume of mitozantrone solution to at least 50 ml in either 0.9% sodium chloride, 5% glucose or 0.18% sodium chloride and 4% glucose.

Bolus administration: Not recommended (mitozantrone must be diluted before administration).

Infusion administration: Mitozantrone infusion should be administered over not less than three minutes via the tubing of a freely-running IV infusion of the above fluids.

Gloves for handling: Latex rubber gloves are recommended.

Extravasation: Mildly irritant. Transient blue discoloration of the tissue will occur but no serious local reaction has been reported.

6 Destruction or Drug or Contaminated Articles

Incineration: 800°C.

Chemical: 5% sodium hydroxide solution/24 hours.

Contact with skin: Wash with water.

References

1. ABPI Data Sheet Compendium 1989/90. (1989). Datapharm Publications Ltd, London, pp. 775–777.
2. Reynolds, D.L. *et al.* (1981). Clinical analysis for the anti-neoplastic agent 1,4-dihydroxy-5,8-bis-2(2-hydroxyethyl)amino) ethyl)-amino. 9,10-anthacenedione dihydrochloride (NSC 301739) in plasma. *J. Chromatography* **222**, 225–240.
3. Trissel, L.A. *et al.* (1985). *Investigational drugs, pharmaceutical data. Pharmaceutical aspects of home infusion therapy for cancer patients.* NCI, Bethesda, Maryland, USA.
4. Adams, P.S. *et al.* (1987). Pharmaceutical aspects of home infusion therapy for cancer patients. *Pharm. J.* **328**, 476–478.
5. Sewell, G.J. *et al.* (1988). Pharmaceutical aspects of domiciliary continuous infusion chemotherapy. *Brit. J. Cancer* **58**, 536.

Prepared by G.J. Sewell

MUSTINE

1 General Details

Approved names: Chlormethine, mustine hydrochloride, mechlorethamine hydrochloride, nitrogen mustard.

Proprietary name: Mustine Hydrochloride.

Manufacturer or supplier: Boots Company Ltd.

Presentation and formulation details: White lyophilized powder in 20 ml vial, containing 10 mg mustine hydrochloride with no excipients.

Storage and shelf-life of unopened container: Two years when stored at 2 to 15°C.

2 Chemistry

Molecular structure: 2-chloro-N-(2-chloroethyl)-N-methyl-ethanamine hydrochloride.

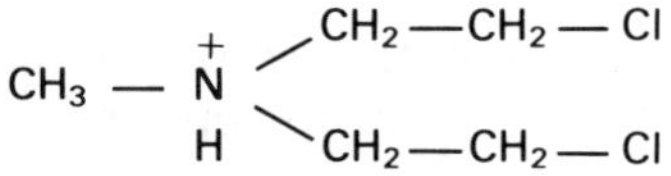

$$CH_3 - \overset{+}{\underset{H}{N}} \Big\langle \begin{matrix} CH_2 - CH_2 - Cl \\ CH_2 - CH_2 - Cl \end{matrix}$$

Molecular weight: 192.5 (hydrochloride).

Solubility: Very soluble in water.

3 Stability Profile

Physical and chemical stability

Degradation pathways: The degradation route of mustine hydrochloride (II) in dilute aqueous solution is shown below:

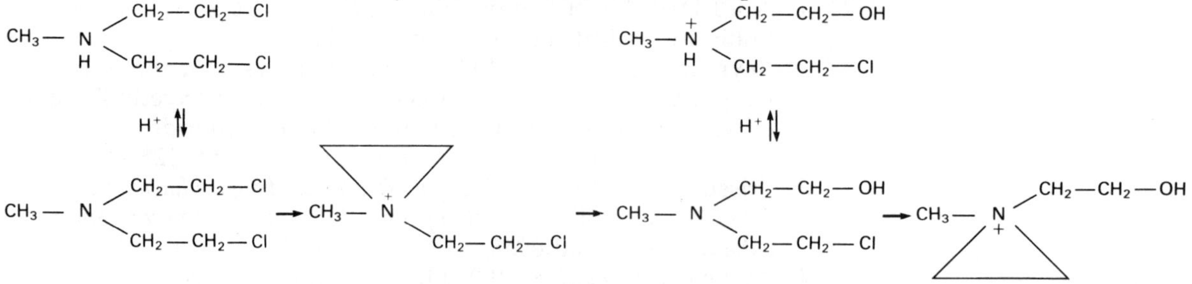

$$(I) \longrightarrow (II) \longrightarrow (III)$$

In aqueous solution mustine appears to lose alkylating activity relatively slowly. Alkylating activity arises from mustine together with compounds II and III in the degradation pathway. However, certain of these degradation products are either more carcinogenic than mustine or may be more neurotoxic.[1,5] Kirk[1] has recently reviewed the conflicting reports in the literature concerning the rate of degradation of mustine in aqueous solution. It is pointed out that almost all studies were carried out using a test for alkylating activity which was not fully stability-indicating. Certain of the products of degradation have alkylating activity *in vitro*. However, an analysis of previous studies indicates that degradation is very pH-dependent,[2] the compound degrading rapidly in neutral or alkaline conditions. An unbuffered solution of mustine has a pH of 3 to 5 and will be more stable. The recent study by Kirk[5] showed that solutions of mustine after reconstitution in 0.9% sodium chloride or water for injections (1 mg/ml) at room temperature, degrade by 8 to 10% in six hours, or by 3 to 6% at 4°C. Solutions diluted in 0.9% sodium chloride (18 to 36 µg/ml) exhibited 15% loss in six hours at room temperature, whilst in 5% glucose, about 11% loss was recorded.

Stability after reconstitution is decreased as the temperature is raised. Mustine is stable in the frozen state (−20°C) for four weeks.[1]

Mustine does not appear to be unduly sensitive to light.

Container compatibility: Kirk[1] has shown recently that mustine does not appear to interact with styrene acrylonitrile syringes (Gillette) or PVC infusion containers.

Compatibility with other drugs: Incompatible with methohexital sodium.[3]

Stability in clinical practice

Reconstituted mustine injection should be used within four hours at room temperature or six hours if stored in the refrigerator.[4] Mustine injection diluted in 500 ml of 0.9% sodium chloride should be administered within two hours, and dilutions in 500 ml of 5% glucose should be used within four hours.[1]

4 Clinical Use

Type of cytotoxic: Alkylating agent.

Main indications: Hodgkin's disease (with other agents).

Dosage: single dose of 0.4 mg/kg body-weight or a course of four daily doses of 0.1 mg/kg body-weight.

5 Preparation of Injection

Reconstitution: To each vial add 10 ml water for injections or 0.9% sodium chloride. The resulting solution contains 1 mg/ml.

Bolus administration: Inject slowly (two minutes) into the bolus site of a fast-running drip of 5% glucose or 0.9% sodium chloride (60 drops/minute).

Infusion: Add the required volume of reconstituted injection to 500 ml of 0.9% sodium chloride injection and infuse slowly over 1 to 2 hours.

Gloves for handling: PVC gloves are recommended.[4] Gloves are essential because mustine is a vesicant and will cause skin blistering.

Extravasation: Very damaging. Antidotes are 3% w/v sodium thiosulphate or 2.5% sodium bicarbonate. Ice compresses are recommended.

6 Destruction of Drug or Contaminated Articles

Incineration: 800°C.

Chemical:

Sodium hydroxide (SG1.5)	1 part) for
IMS	4 parts) 48
Water	3 parts) hours.

Contact with skin: Wash immediately with large amounts of water. Can be neutralized with sodium thiosulphate or sodium bicarbonate.

References

1. Kirk, B. (1986). Stability of reconstituted mustine injection BP during storage. *Brit. J. Parent. Therap.* **7**, 86–92.
2. Friedman, O.M. and Boger, E. (1961). Colorimetric estimation of nitrogen mustards in aqueous media. *Analytical Chem.* **33**, 907–910.
3. Trissel, L.A. (1988). *Handbook of injectable drugs*, 5nd edn, American Society of Hospital Pharmacists, Bethesda, Maryland, USA.
4. ABPI Datasheet Compendium 1989/1990. (1989). Datapharm Publications Ltd, London, pp. 231–232.
5. Kirk, B. (1987). A study of the stability of aqueous solutions of mustine hydrochloride using colorimetric and HPLC assay techniques. *Proc. of Guild.* **23**, 47–52.

Prepared by M.C. Allwood

THIOTEPA

1 General Details

Approved names: Thiotepa, thiophosphoramide, TESPA, TSPA.

Proprietary name: Thiotepa.

Manufacturer or supplier: Lederle Laboratories Ltd.

Presentation and formulation details: Lyophilized powder, in vials containing thiotepa 15 mg, sodium chloride 80 mg and sodium bicarbonate 50 mg.

Storage and shelf-life of unopened container: The injection has a shelf-life of three years, when stored between 2 to 8°C.

2 Chemistry

Molecular structure: 1,1'1″-phosphinothioyldinetris-aziridine.

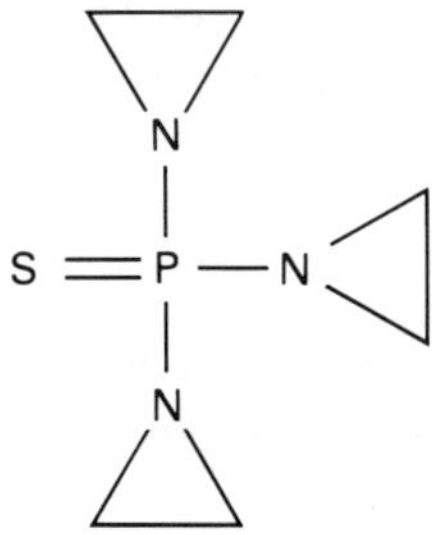

Molecular weight: 189.2.

Solubility: Soluble 1 in 8 in water; 1 in 2 in ethanol; 1 in 2 in chloroform; and 1 in 4 ether.

3 Stability Profile

Physical and chemical stability

The stability of thiotepa in aqueous solution is pH-dependent; it is least stable in acid solutions. The acid catalysed reaction of thiotepa in the presence of chloride ions yields a series of chloroethyl derivatives (I-III) according to the following scheme:[1]

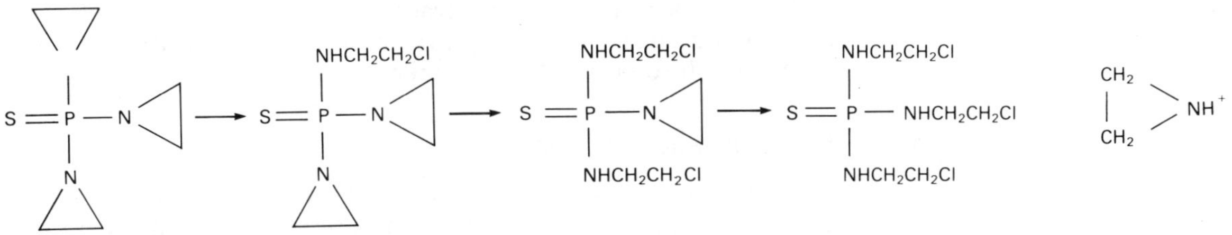

(I) → (II) → (III) → (IV)

In strong acid solutions and in aqueous solutions at elevated temperatures, thiotepa undergoes P-N cleavage and/or ring-opening to give the azaridinium ion (IV).[2] Thiotepa will also polymerize to form insoluble polymeric derivatives.

At 37°C in pH 4.2 buffer the rate constant for loss of thiotepa is 9.8×10^{-3} minute^{-1} giving a $t^{90\%}$ of 10 minutes. At pH 7 degradation was much slower; no breakdown could be detected after two hours at 37°C but longer term data were not available.[3]

Any polymerization reaction is likely to be catalysed by light, reducing the stability of thiotepa.

Stability in clinical practice

The reconstituted solution has a shelf-life of five days when stored at 2 to 8°C.[4] A 0.05% solution retains 88% of potency after storage at 3°C for 35 days.[5] Solutions of 0.25 mg/ml in normal saline are stable for seven days at 25°C in PVC bags.[6]

When administered as a bladder irrigation it is recommended that up to 60 mg thiotepa in 60 ml sterile water is instilled and the solution retained in the bladder for up to two hours. Thiotepa is, however, unstable in acidic urine at 37°C. At pH 5.5, $t_{90\%}$ is 70 minutes and, at pH 4.0, $t_{90\%}$ is 3.3 minutes with only 2.1% of the initial dose of thiotepa remaining after two hours.[3] The irrigation solution contains 200 mg sodium bicarbonate which should maintain sufficiently alkaline conditions in the bladder, but large volumes of acidic urine may present problems.

4 Clinical Use

Type of cytotoxic: Thiotepa is a polyfunctional alkylating agent. It releases ethylenimine radicals which disrupt the bonds of DNA.

Main indications: Adenocarcinoma of the breast and of the ovary; for controlling intracavity effusions secondary to diffuse or localized neoplastic disease of various serosal cavities; and for the treatment of superficial papalliary carcinoma of the bladder.[5] Thiotepa has been effective against lymphosarcoma and Hodgkin's disease but is now largely superseded by other treatments. It has been used also for the post-operative management of pterygium.[7,8]

Dosage: By rapid intravenous infusion, 0.3 to 0.4 mg/kg at one to four week intervals. By intracavity instillation, 10 to 65 mg in 20 to 60 ml sterile water. By intravesical administration, up to 60 mg in 30 to 60 ml sterile water.

5 Preparation of Injection

Reconstitution: Reconstitution of the 15 mg vial with 1.5 ml water gives a 10 mg/ml solution. If the thiotepa has polymerized a precipitate will form on reconstitution. Precipitated solutions should be discarded.

Administration: For intracavity instillation first aspirate as much fluid as possible then instil the dose of thiotepa. The same tubing may be used for both aspiration and instillation.

For bladder instillation the patient is dehydrated for eight to 12 hours. The solution is instilled into the bladder and retained there for two hours.

Gloves for handling: Both PVC and latex are permeable to thiotepa at a concentration of 10 mg/ml within 90 minutes.[9] Latex surgeons' gloves should be used and the gloves should be changed every 30 minutes.

Extravasation: Thiotepa is nonvesicant and non-irritant.

6 Destruction of Drug or Contaminated Articles

Incineration: 800°C.

Chemical: Dilute in large quantities of boiling water.

Contact with skin: Wash off with water.

References

1. Maxwell, J. *et al.* (1974). Behaviour of an aziridine alkylating agent in acid solution. *Biochem. Pharmacol.* **23**, 168–170.
2. Zon, G. *et al.* (1976). Observations of 1,1',1'' phosphino-thioylidinetrisaziridine (thiotepa) in acidic and saline media. An[1] H-NRM study. *Biochem. Pharmacol.* **25**, 989–992.
3. Cohen, G.E. *et al.* (1984). Effects of pH and temperature on the stability and decomposition of N,N'N'' triethylenethio-phosphoramide in urine and buffer. *Cancer Res.* **44**, 4312–4316.
4. Kirschembaum, B.E. and Latiolais, C.J. (1976). Stability of injectable medications after reconstitution. *Am. J. Hosp. Pharm.* **33**, 767–791.
5. Personal communication, Manufacturer's Data.
6. Uyas, H.M. *et al.* (1987). Drug stability guidelines for a continuous infusion chemotherapy programme. *Hosp. Pharm.* **22**, 685–687.
7. Erlich, D. (1977). The management of pterygium. *Ophth. Surg.* **8**, 23–30.
8. Olander, K. (1978). Management of pterygium: should thiotepa be used? *Ann. Ophthalmol.* **10**, 853–856.
9. Laidlaw, J.L. *et al.* (1984) Permeability of latex and poly-vinylchloride gloves to 20 antineoplastic drugs. *Am. J. Hosp. Pharm.* **41**, 2618–2623.

Prepared by M.G. Lee

VINBLASTINE

1 General Details

Approved names: Vinblastine, vincaleukoblastine.

Proprietary name: Velbe (Lilly).

Manufacturers or suppliers: Eli Lilly & Co. Ltd, Lederle Laboratories Ltd, David Bull Laboratories Ltd (DBL).

Presentation and formulation details: Lyophilized powder containing 10 mg vinblastine sulphate. This is supplied with 10 ml aqueous diluent containing 90 mg sodium chloride and 0.2 ml benzyl alcohol (Lilly, Lederle, DBL).

Storage and shelf-life of unopened container: The injection has a shelf-life of three years when stored between 0 and 6°C.

2. Chemistry

Type: Vinca alkaloid.

Molecular Structure: Vincaleucoblastine.

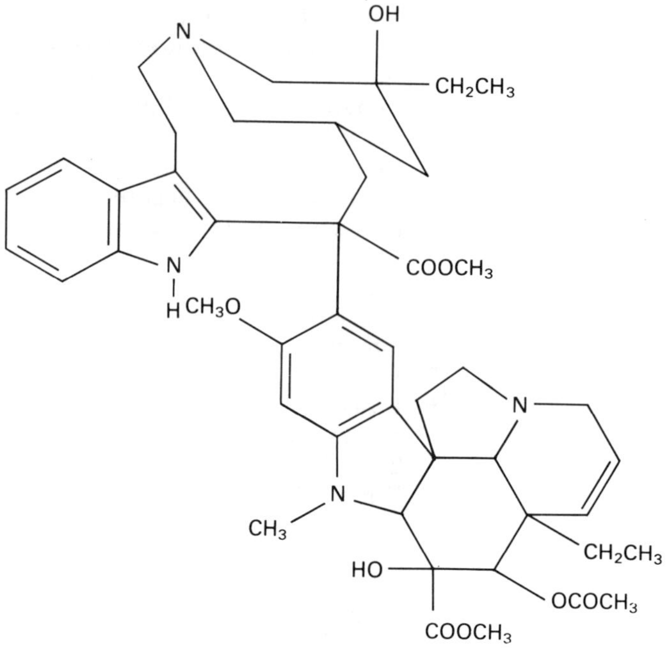

Molecular weight: 811.0 (vinblastine sulphate: 909.0).

Solubility: The base is insoluble in water; soluble in ethanol and chloroform. The sulphate salt is soluble 1 in 10 water; 1 in 1200 ethanol; 1 in 50 chloroform. pKa: 5.4, 7.4.

3 Stability Profile

Physical and chemical stability

Degradation pathways: Aqueous solutions of vinblastine are less stable at lower pH values, 4-desacetylvinblastine is the primary degradation product at pH 2.[1] More recent studies indicate that the hydrolytic decomposition pathways for vinblastine are more complex. Below pH 1.5 and above pH 10.5, desacetylvinblastine has been confirmed as the major degradation product. However, between pH 2.5 and 7.0, the amount of desacetylvinblastine found was negligible and at least three other degradation products were detected.[2] Studies on 1 mg/ml solutions of vinblastine sulphate at pH 4.5 to 5.0 identified up to six breakdown products. The major degradents were tentatively identified as 19′-oxo-vinblastine and an isomer of vinblastine but none of the decomposition products were positively categorized. From the data at 25, 37 and 55°C, $t^{90\%}$'s were estimated to be 16.6 days at 37°C, 150 days at 25°C and 10.7 years at 5°C.[3]

When exposed to direct incandescent light, decomposition is accelerated. At 25°C, the $t^{90\%}$ is approximately seven days and at 30°C, solutions of vinblastine sulphate had lost 10% of their potency after slightly more than one day.[4] The major degradation products were different from those identified in thermal degradation studies but the same pattern of products were identified in both cases.

Vinblastine base is practically insoluble in water and can precipitate from solutions of vinblastine sulphate above pH 6.

Container compatibility: No loss of potency was detected from solutions of vinblastine sulphate (10 mg/ml) stored for 30 days in polypropylene syringes at 4°C or room temperature.[5] There was no significant loss of potency when vinblastine sulphate solution 10 mg in 50 ml in 5% glucose or 0.9% sodium chloride was filtered through a 0.22 µm cellulose ester membrane filter.[6]

Losses of 24% occurred in 24 hours at 37°C from a 1 mg/ml solution of vinblastine sulphate in bacteriostatic 0.9% saline in an Infusaid implantable pump; in 12 days losses totalled 48%. Similar solutions in glass vials exhibited no losses after 24 hours and 20% loss after 12 days at 37°C.[7]

Vinblastine has been shown to be absorbed on to PVC tubing and cellulose proprionate burette chambers. Up to 48% loss was found from a 3 µg/ml solution stored for 48 hours in PVC tubing and up to 20% loss of potency was found in similar solutions stored in cellulose proprionate burette chambers for 48 hours.[8] These results were obtained for a static system and it is difficult to extrapolate them to the dynamic situation of an intravenous administration. Significant losses are likely to occur, however, in PVC administration sets. The absorption losses did not occur in polybutadiene tubing or methacrylate butadiene styrene burettes.[8]

Stability in clinical practice

The reconstituted injection is chemically stable for at least 28 days at 4°C and at 25°C,[3] provided it is protected from light. When stored at 37°C in the dark, the shelf-life of the reconstituted injection is 14 days. In direct incandescent light, the injection is chemically stable for 7 days at room temperature.[4]

4 Clinical Use

Type of cytotoxic: Vinblastine arrests mitosis at the metaphase and inhibits RNA synthesis.

Main indications: Vinblastine is used in combination with other chemotherapeutic agents for treatment of metastatic testicular carcinoma, Hodgkin's and non-Hodgkin's lymphoma, neuroblastoma, histiocytosis X, mycosis fungoides, Kaposi's sarcoma, advanced breast carcinoma and choriocarcinoma.

Dosage: Usually 4 to 8 mg/m² weekly. Weekly injections starting at 3.7 mg/m² and rising by increments of 1.85 mg/m² up to a maximum of 18.5 mg/m² or until the white cell count has fallen to 3000/mm³ have been used.[9]

5 Preparation of Injection

Reconstitution: Reconstitution of the 10 mg vial with 10 ml of sterile diluent gives a 1 mg/ml solution.

Administration: Intravenously, directly into vein or into the tubing of a running infusion, over a one-minute period. Vinblastine has also been given as a continuous five-day infusion (1.4 to 2.0 mg/m^2/day[10]). Infusions should be administered through a central line.

Constant ambulatory intravenous infusion has been investigated using a tunnelled subclavian catheter and the Cor-med ML6 infusion pump[11] and the Travenol Infuser system.[12] There are, however, insufficient data to draw reliable conclusions from this work.

Gloves for handling: Latex rubber gloves are recommended.

Extravasation: Moderate to severe. Hyaluronidase 1000 units diluted ten times in normal saline may be useful.

6 Destruction of Drug or Contaminated Articles

Incineration: 1000°C.

Chemical: Hot water.

Contact with skin: Wash with copious amounts of water.

References

1. Burns, J.H. (1972). *Analytical profiles of drug substance*, Vol. 1, Academic Press, Orlando, Florida, USA, pp. 443.
2. Vendrig, D.E.M.M. *et al.* (1988). Degradation kinetics of vinblastine sulphate in aqueous solutions. *Int. J. Pharm.* **43**, 131–138.
3. Black, J. *et al.* (1988). Studies on the stability of vinblastine sulphate in aqueous solution. *J. Pharm. Sci.* **77**, 630.
4. Black, J. *et al.* (1988). Stability of vinblastine sulphate when exposed to light. *Drug Intell. Clin. Pharm.* **22**, 634.
5. Ireland, D. *et al.* (1990). The chemical stability of cytarabine and vinblastine injections. *Br. J. Pharm. Pract.* **12**, 53–54.
6. Butler, L.D. *et al.* (1980). Effect of in-line filtration on the potency of low-dose drugs. *Am. J. Hosp. Pharm.* **37**, 935.
7. Keller, J.H. and Ensminger, W.D. (1982). Stability of cancer chemotherapeutic agents in totally implanted drug delivery systems. *Am. J. Hosp. Pharm.* **39**, 1321.
8. McElany, J.C. *et al.* (1988). Stability of methotrexate and vinblastine in burette administration sets. *Int. J. Pharm.* **47**, 239–247.
9. Anon. (1986). *Physicians desk reference*, 40th edn, Medical Economics Company, Oradell, New Jersey, USA.
10. Yap, H.Y. *et al.* (1980). Vinblastine given as a continuous five-day infusion in the treatment of refractory advanced breast cancer. *Cancer Treat. Rep.* **64**, 279.
11. Lokich, J. *et al.* (1982). The delivery of cancer chemotherapy by constant venous infusion. *Cancer* **50**, 2731.

12. Akokoshi, M.P. *et al.* (1987). Safety and reliability of the Travenol Infusor, *J. Pharm. Technol.* (Mar/Apr), 65.

Prepared by M.G. Lee

VINCRISTINE

1 General Details

Approved names: Vincristine, leurocristine.

Proprietary name: Oncovin (Lilly).

Manufacturers or suppliers: David Bull Laboratories Ltd (DBL), Eli Lilly & Co. Ltd, Lederle Laboratories Ltd.

Presentation and formulation details: Lyophilized powder containing lactose in the following proportions of vincristine to lactose: 1 mg–10 mg, 2 mg–20 mg, 5 mg–50 mg. Supplied with 10 ml of diluent containing 90 mg sodium chloride and 0.2 ml benzyl alcohol (Lilly, Lederle, DBL).

1 ml and 2 ml vials containing vincristine sulphate 1 mg/ml in solution with mannitol 100 mg/ml, methylhydroxybenzoate 1.8 mg/ml and propylhydroxybenzoate 0.2 mg/ml (Lilly), or preservative-free (DBL); also available in prefilled syringes (DBL).

Storage and shelf-life of unopened containers: When stored at 0 to 6°C, the lyophilized powder has a shelf-life of three years and the solution has a shelf-life of two years.

2 Chemistry

Type: Vinca alkaloid.

Molecular structure: 22-oxo-Vincaleukoblastine (sulphate salt).

Molecular weight: 825.1 (Vincristine sulphate: 923).

Solubility: Sulphate salt: 1 in 2 of water; 1 in 600 of ethanol; 1 in 30 of chloroform. pKa: 5.0, 7.4.

3 Stability Profile

Physical and chemical stability

Vincristine is hydrolyzed in aqueous solution to the desacetyl derivative. Kinetic data are not available for this reaction but since the injection solution has a shelf-life of 18 months when stored at 0 to 6°C, solutions with a pH of 3.5 to 5.5 would be expected to be equally stable.

Vincristine base is insoluble in water and so vincristine sulphate solutions can precipitate above pH 6.

Effect of light: No problems with degradation due to light have been reported.

Container compatibility: No losses to plastic (PVC) containers or syringes have been reported.

After filtration through a 0.22 μm cellulose ester filter, 6.5% of a 1 mg/50 ml solution in 5% glucose and 12% of a 1 mg/50 ml solution in 0.9% sodium chloride was bound to the filter.[2] Vincristine sulphate, 1.5 mg in 3 ml, when injected as a bolus through a 0.22 μm nylon filter and after flushing the filter with 10 ml normal saline, showed losses of 10% of the vincristine to the filter.[3]

Stability in clinical practice

The reconstituted injection is chemically stable for 30 days when stored at 2 to 6°C, and the diluted infusion solution is equally stable. The solution is compatible with PVC containers and plastic syringes.

The injection solution is stable for 18 months when stored under refrigeration and for at least one month at room temperature.[4]

4 Clinical Use

Type of cytotoxic: Vincristine blocks mitosis with metaphase arrest by binding to tubulin and inhibiting the assembly of microtubules. It is M-phase specific.

Main indications: Vincristine is used, principally in combination chemotherapy regimens, against Hodgkin's and non-Hodgkin's lymphomas, acute lymphocytic leukaemia, lymphosarcoma, reticulum cell sarcoma, rhabdomyosarcoma, neuroblastoma, Wilm's tumour, advanced breast carcinoma and small-cell lung carcinoma. It has modest to moderate activity in many other malignancies.[5]

Dosage: 1.4 mg/m^2 weekly, up to a maximum of 2 mg. In children weighing less than 10 kg, 0.05 mg/kg weekly is used. Due to the narrow therapeutic range, the dose should be individually adjusted.

5 Preparation of Injection

Reconstitution: Add 1 ml of diluent to a 1 mg vial, 2 ml to a 2 mg vial and 5 ml to a 5 mg vial to give a 1 mg/ml solution.

Bolus administration: By bolus injection or into the tubing of a running intravenous infusion. As it is vesicant, care must be taken to avoid extravasation during administration. Vincristine has also been administered by continuous infusion[5] with reported higher blood concentrations and increased tumour response at a dose of 0.5 mg/m^2 daily for five days in three-week cycles.[6]

Gloves for handling: Latex rubber gloves are recommended.

Extravasation: Moderate to severe. 1000 units of hyaluronidase in 20 ml normal saline may aid recovery.

6 Destruction of Drugs or Contaminated Articles

Incineration: 1000°C.

Chemical: 5% sodium hypochlorite/24 hours.

Contact with skin: Wash with copious amounts of water.

References

1. ABPI Data Sheet Compendium 1989/90. (1989). Datapharm Publications Ltd, London, pp. 785–786, 845–846.
2. Butler, L.D. *et al.* (1980). Effect of in-line filtration on the potency of low-dose drugs. *Am. J. Hosp. Pharm.* **37**, 935–941.
3. Ennis, C.E. *et al.* (1983). *In vitro* study of in-line filtration of medications commonly administered to paediatric cancer patients. *J. Parent. Enter. Nutrit.* 7, 156–158.
4. Vegenbery, F.R. and Souney, P.F. (1983). Stability guidelines for routinely refrigerated drug products. *Am. J. Hosp. Pharm.* **40**, 101–102.
5. Smith, B.D. Antitumour update: Vinca alkaloids and epipodophyllotoxins. *Hosp. Formul.* **22**, 363–373.
6. Jackson, D.V. *et al.* (1984). Intravenous vincristine infusion. *Cancer,* **48**, 2559–2664.
7. Jackson, D.V. *et al.* (1981) Pharmacokinetics of vincristine infusion. *Cancer Treat. Rep.* **65**, 1043–1048.

Prepared by M.G. Lee

VINDESINE

1 General Details

Approved names: Vindesine, desacetyl vinblastine amide.

Proprietary name: Eldisine.

Manufacturer or supplier: Eli Lilly & Co. Ltd.

Presentation and formulation details: Lyophilized powder consisting of 5 mg vindesine sulphate with 25 mg mannitol. Supplied with 5 ml sterile diluent containing sodium chloride 9 mg/ml and 2% benzyl alcohol adjusted to pH 4.2 to 4.5 with hydrochloric acid or sodium hydroxide.[1]

Storage and shelf-life of unopened container: When stored between 2 and 6°C, the injection has a shelf-life of three years.

2 Chemistry

Type: Vinca alkaloid and synthetic derivative of vinblastine.

Molecular structure: 3-(aminocarbonyl)-O-deacetyl-3-de(methoxycarbonyl)-Vincaleukoblastine.

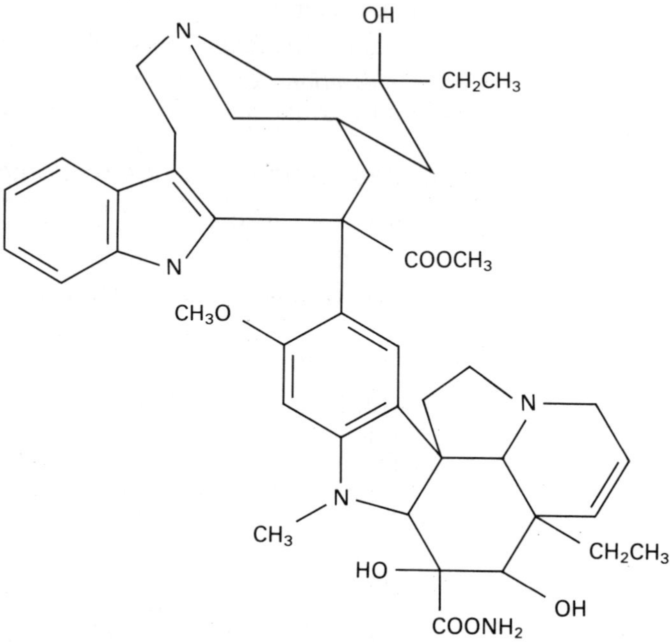

Molecular weight: 753.9 (Vindesine sulphate: 852).

Solubility: The sulphate salt is freely soluble in water. pKa: 5.4, 7.4.

3 Stability Profile

Physical and chemical stability

Unlike the naturally occurring vinca alkaloids, vindesine does not possess an acetyl group at the 4-position and is therefore less prone to hydrolysis than vincristine and vinblastine.

Aqueous solutions of vindesine are chemically stable for 30 days when stored at 0–6°C.[1]

The reconstituted injection has a pH of 4.2 to 4.5. Precipitation will occur above pH 6.

Stability in clinical practice

The reconstituted injection and diluted infusion solutions are chemically stable for at least 30 days.[1] Vindesine solutions are compatible with PVC containers and plastic syringes.

4 Clinical Use

Type of cytotoxic: Vindesine causes metaphase arrest by binding to tubulin, a substructure of the microtubular spindle apparatus. This leads to inhibition of tubulin polymerization which interrupts mitosis and leads to cell death.[2] For a complete review of the antineoplastic activity of vindesine see Cersosima *et al.*[2]

Main indications: Acute lymphoblastic leukaemia, chronic myelogenous leukaemia in blast crisis, malignant melanoma and advanced breast carcinoma.

Dosage: 3 to 4 mg/m^2 weekly as a bolus injection, or by four hour[3] or 48 hour infusion.[4] For fuller details of dosage regimens see Cersosima *et al.*[2]

5 Preparation of Injection

Reconstitution: Reconstitute the 5 mg vial with 5 ml of sterile diluent to give a 1 mg/ml solution.

Administration: Intravenous infusions of the drug should be prepared in glucose or sodium chloride solutions. Multi-electrolyte infusion solutions such as lactated Ringer's should not be used because of the possibility of precipitation of the drug.

Gloves for handling: Latex rubber gloves are recommended.

Extravasation: Moderate to severe. 1000 units of hyaluronidase in 20 ml saline may aid recovery.

6 Destruction of Drug or Contaminated Articles

Incineration: 1000°C.

Chemical: 5% sodium hypochlorite/24 hours.

Contact with skin: Wash with copious amounts of water.

References

1. ABPI Data Sheet Compendium 1989/1990. (1989). Datapharm Publications Ltd, London, pp. 828–829.
2. Cersosima, R.J. *et al.* (1983). Pharmacology, clinical efficacy and adverse effects of vindesine sulphate, a new vinca alkaloid. *Pharmacotherapy* **3**, 259–268.
3. Ettinger, L.J. *et al.* (1982). Vindesine – phase II study in childhood malignancies – a report for cancer and leukaemia group. *Br. Med. Pediatr. Oncol.* **10**, 35–44.
4. Mathe, G. *et al.* (1981). Phase II clinical trials with haematogical malignancies. *Anticancer Res.* **1**, 1–10.

Prepared by M.G. Lee

This section provides and identifies suitable sources of essential basic information on unlicensed cytotoxic agents known to be of current clinical interest. The interferons, interleukins and related biologically-derived compounds, now all known generically as cytokines, have been intentionally excluded since they do not present to pharmacy staff the same problems of handling as do more conventional cytotoxic agents.

Much of the content draws heavily on information provided by the National Cancer Institute (NCI) of the National Institute of Health of the USA. Copies of two books, *NCI investigational drugs: pharmaceutical data* and *Investigational drugs: chemical data*, which are updated annually, may be obtained by post, free of charge from:

Pharmaceutical Resources Branch
National Cancer Institute
Executive Plaza North
Suite 818
Bethesda, Maryland 20892
USA.

More comprehensive information may also be available from the NCI in clinical brochures for individual drugs, or from investigators currently working with the compounds concerned. For this reason, at the end of each monograph, UK centres with a known interest in the compound concerned are identified.

BISANTRENE

1 General Details

Approved name: Bisantrene.

Proprietary name: Cyabin.

Manufacturer or supplier: Cyanamid (USA).

Presentation and formulation details: Vials containing 50 mg, 250 mg or 500 mg of lyophilized bisantrene. Contains no excipients.

Storage and shelf-life of unopened containers: Unreconstituted vials should be stored at room temperature, protected from light and have a 5-year shelf-life.

2 Chemistry

Type: Anthracene.

Molecular structure: 9,10-anthracenedicarboxaldehyde bis (4,5-dihydro-1H-imidazol-2-yl) hydrozone dihydrochloride.

Molecular weight: 471.4.

Solubility: Soluble in water.

3 Stability profile

Infusions of bisantrene at a concentration of 0.5 mg/ml should be used within 4 hours of preparation.

Compatibility: A 25 mg/ml solution should be prepared in water for injection only. Subsequent dilution should be in 5% glucose or 0.9% sodium chloride.

4 Clinical Use

Main indications: Treatment of acute leukaemias

5 Preparation of Injection

Reconstitution: The 50 mg, 250 mg, 500 mg strength vials of bisantrene should be reconstituted to a clear solution by adding 2 ml, 10 ml and 20 ml respectively, of water for injections. Avoid, for solubility reasons, any other parenteral diluents.

Filter needles should not be used for reconstituting bisantrene. Instead, change the needle (preferably to a smaller size) prior to injecting into the IV bag or bottle.

Dilution: The reconstituted solution (25 mg/ml) should then be diluted to a final concentration of 0.5 mg/ml by slow addition of the reconstituted solution to appropriate volumes of 5% glucose or 0.9% sodium chloride. Dilution below 0.5 mg/ml is not recommended. The diluted solution should be administered within four hours, protecting from exposure to intense light or sunlight by covering the IV bag or bottle with aluminium foil or light-protecting overwrap.

Administration: IV infusion over 2 hours.

Gloves for handling: PVC gloves are recommended.

Extravasation: The drug is extremely vesicant.

6 Destruction of Drug or Contaminated Articles

Incineration: No information.

Chemical: Use an aqueous solution of calcium hydroxide (5.5 parts calcium hydroxide in 13 parts by weight of water for each 1 part of bisantrene). Absorb the solution with gauze or towels and dispose of these in a safe manner.

Contact with skin: Experimental animal studies have revealed that bisantrene, in powder or solution form, has the potential to produce moderate to severe ocular irritation, mild skin irritation or contact sensitization. Therefore, if the powder or solution of bisantrene comes into accidental contact with the skin of an individual, thoroughly wash the exposed area with soap and warm water. Rinse copiously with warm (not hot) water. If there is accidental contact with the eyes, flush affected eye(s) with copious amounts of water for at least 15 minutes while holding the eyelid(s) open. Obtain appropriate medical assistance, including ophthalmological consultation for follow-up and monitoring.

7 UK Centres with a Known Interest in this Drug

University Hospital of Wales, Cardiff.

8 Sources of Information

Pharmacy Brochure prepared by Medical Research Division, American Cyanamid Company, August 1986.

Prepared by T. Root

DEOXYCOFORMYCIN

1 General Details

Approved names: Deoxycoformycin, 2-deoxycoformycin, co-vidarabine, pentostatin.

Proprietary names: None.

Manufacturer or supplier: National Cancer Institute.

Presentation and formulation details: Vials of white lyophilized powder containing 10 mg deoxycoformycin. Each vial also contains 50 mg mannitol and sodium hydroxide to adjust pH.

Storage and shelf-life of unopened containers: Store at 2 to 8°C. Vials are labelled with an expiry date.

2 Chemistry

Type: Antimetabolite.

Molecular structure: Imidazo (4,5-d d)(1,3)diazepin-8-ol, 3-(1-dexoy-beta-D-erythro-pentafuranoesyl)-3,4,7.8-tetrahydro-

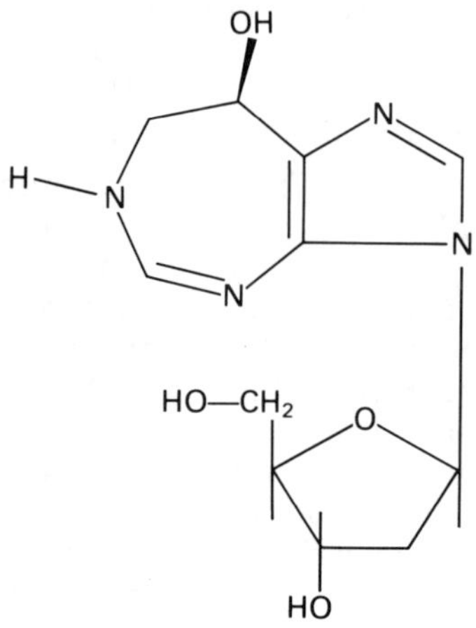

Molecular weight: 268.3.

Solubility: Greater than 30 mg/ml in water.

3 Stability Profile

Physical and chemical stability: Constitution with 0.9% sodium chloride, results in a solution which is chemically stable at room temperature (22 to 25°C) for at least 72 hours exhibiting about 2 to 4% decomposition.

Effect of temperature: When diluted to a concentration of 10 mg in 500 ml 0.9% sodium chloride, or lactated Ringer's Injection, deoxycoformycin is chemically stable for at least 48 hours at room temperature (22 to 25°C), exhibiting less than 5% decomposition.

At a concentration of 10 mg per 500 ml in 5% glucose, approximately 2% decomposition occurs in 24 hours at room temperature. As much as 8 to 10% loss has been reported to occur in 48 hours.

No potency loss was detected in this reconstituted solution or in admixtures in 5% glucose or 0.9% sodium chloride, when refrigerated at 5°C over 96 hours.

4 Clinical Use

Main indications: Treatment of hairy cell leukaemia, chronic lymphocytic leukaemia.

5 Preparation of Injection

Reconstitution: 5 ml of 0.9% sodium chloride is added to provide a solution containing deoxycoformycin 2 mg/ml which has a pH of 6.7 to 8.7.

Bolus administration: IV bolus, slowly over 3 to 5 minutes.

Gloves for handling: Latex gloves are suggested.

Extravasation: The solution is non-irritant.

6 Destruction of Drug or Contaminated Articles

Incineration: No specific information.
Chemical: No specific information.
Contact with skin: No specific information.

7 UK Centres with a Known Interest in this Drug

The Royal Marsden Hospital, Hammersmith Hospital.

8 Source of Information

NCI investigational drug data, 1989

Prepared by T. Root

FLUDARABINE

1 General Details

Approved names: Fludarabine, fludarabine phosphate, 2-fluoro-adrenine arabinoside-5-phosphate, 2-fluoro-ARA-AMP.
Proprietary names: None.
Manufacturer or supplier: National Cancer Institute. Fludarabine is also manufactured for Triton Biosciences Inc, Alameda, California 94501, USA and by Ben Venue Labs Inc. Bedford, Ohio 44146, USA.
Presentation and formulation details: 5 ml vials of white lyophilized powder containing 50 mg fludarabine. Each vial also contains mannitol 50 mg and sodium hydroxide to adjust pH.
Storage and shelf-life of unopened containers: Store at 2 to 8°C (NCI) or at 15 to 30°C (Triton).

2 Chemistry

Type: Antimetabolite.
Molecular structure: 9H-Purine-6-amine, 2-fluoro-9-(5-o-phosphono-B-D-arabinofuranoeyl).

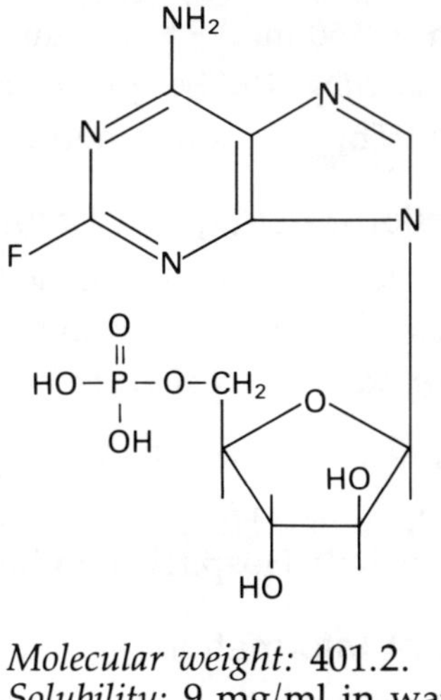

Molecular weight: 401.2.
Solubility: 9 mg/ml in water.

3 Stability Profile

Physical and chemical stability

Shelf-life surveillance of the intact vials is ongoing. One lot has maintained stability after 36 months at room temperature (22 to 25°C) and under refrigeration (2 to 8°C).

Effect of pH: Fludarabine phosphate is relatively stable in aqueous solution. Over a pH range of approximately 4.5 to 8 in aqueous buffer solutions stored at 65°C, less than 4% decomposition occurred in 1 day and less than 10% occurred in 4 days. At pH 3 at 65°C, approximately 11% decomposition occurred in 1 day. From this pH profile, the optimum pH was determined to be approximately 7.6.

Effect of temperature: At a concentration of 25 mg/ml in distilled water stored at room temperature (22 to 25°C) in normal laboratory light, fludarabine phosphate exhibited less than 2% decomposition in 16 days.

Diluted to a concentration of 1 mg/ml in 5% glucose or in 0.9% sodium chloride, less than 3% decomposition occurred in 16 days at room temperature (22 to 25°C) under normal laboratory light.

Diluted to a concentration of 0.0 4 mg/ml in 5% glucose or in 0.9% sodium chloride in glass bottles and PVC bags, little or no loss occurred in 48 hours at room temperature (22 to 25°C) exposed to normal laboratory light and under refrigeration (about 5°C).

4 Clinical Use

Main indications: Treatment of non-Hodgkin's lymphoma, chronic lymphoblastic leukaemia.

5 Preparation of Injection

Reconstitution: 2 ml of water for injection is added to a 50 mg vial to give a solution of pH 6.5 to 8.5 containing 25 mg fludarabine, 25 mg mannitol and sodium hydroxide.

Bolus administration: Slow bolus in 10 ml 0.9% sodium chloride or infusion in 250 ml 0.9% sodium chloride.

Gloves for handling: Rubber gloves are suggested.

Extravastion: The solution is non-irritant.

6 Destruction of Drug or Contaminated Articles

Incineration: No specific information.

Chemical: No specific information.

Contact with skin: No specific information.

7 UK Centres with a Known Interest in this Drug

The Royal Marsden Hospital, London
St Bartholomew's Hospital, London.

8 Source of Information

NCI investigational drug data, 1989.

Prepared by T. Root

STREPTOZOCIN

1 General details

Approved name: Streptozocin.

Proprietary name: Zanosar.

Manufacturer or supplier: Upjohn (UK) Limited.

Presentation and formulation details: Pale-yellow freeze-dried powder containing 1 g streptozocin. Contains sodium hydroxide to adjust pH. Each vial also contains 220 mg citric acid. Contains no preservatives.

Storage and shelf-life of unopened containers: Store at 2 to 8°C, protected from light.

2. Chemistry

Type: Nitrosurea.

Molecular structure: 2-deoxy-2-(methyl-nitrosoamino)carbonylamino-(and B)-D-glucopyranose.

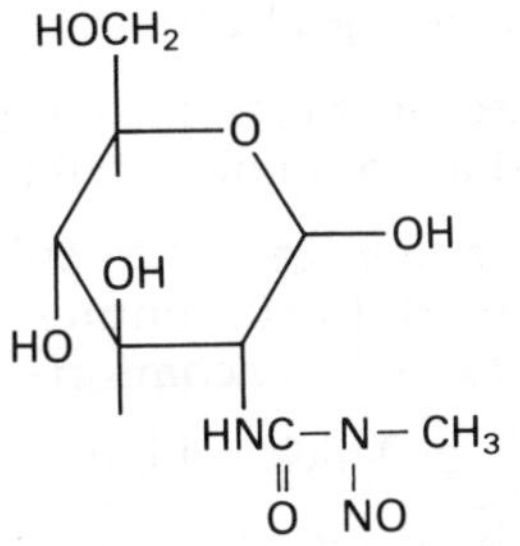

Molecular weight: 265.2.

Solubility: Soluble in water, 0.9% sodium chloride and ethanol.

3 Stability Profile

Physical and chemical stability

Effect of temperature: Streptozocin was reconstituted in 1 L of 20% glucose. The final concentration of the solution was 1 mg/ml. The study indicated a less than 10% degradation after 72 hours at both 5°C and 22 to 24°C.

The injection was stable for more than 60 hours at 4 and 25°C when reconstituted with water for injection or 0.9% sodium chloride.

1 g vials were reconstituted with 9.5 ml of 0.9% sodium chloride irrigation, 20% glucose, and deionized water. The vials were stored at 3 and 24°C. pH fell slightly after 48 hours at 24°C, consistent with initial degradation of streptozocin. All

solutions were clear, pale-yellow at reconstitution and no colour changes were discernible over 48 hours. No particulates or cloudiness observed in the vials.

Effect of light: A significant loss of potency was observed after 340 days and 740 days of exposure to light.

The freeze-dried product, when stored under conditions of minimal light exposure, did not show significant potency reduction.

Compatibility: Streptozocin may be reconstituted in water for injections 0.9% sodium chloride or 5% glucose.

Container compatibility: Vials containing 1 g of streptozocin were reconstituted with 9.5 ml of 5% glucose or 0.9%. Sodium chloride aliquots of 10 ml were transferred to 1 L plastic IV bags (Abbott). Samples were assayed for DEHP over a 48-hour period. No leeching of DEHP from the plastic into the streptozocin solution was observed.

4 Clinical use

Main indications: Metastatic islet cell tumours of the pancreas.

5 Preparation of Injection

Reconstitution: Reconstitute each 1 g vial with 9.5 ml of diluent to yield a solution containing 100 mg/ml streptozocin.

Infusion administration: In 250 to 500 ml 0.9% sodium chloride or 5% glucose; over 30 to 60 minutes. Bolus not recommended because it is extremely uncomfortable for the patient.

Gloves for handling: Thick rubber latex recommended.

Extravasation: The drug solution is vesicant. No specific recommendations for management.

6 Destruction of Drug or Contaminated Articles

Incineration: No specific information.
Chemical: No specific information.
Contact with the skin: No specific information.

7 UK Centres with a Known Interest in this Drug

The Royal Marsden Hospital, London.
Hammersmith Hospital, London.

8 Source of Information

Personal communication from Upjohn (UK) Ltd. February 1990. Zanosar Data Sheet.

Prepared by T. Root

TENIPOSIDE

1 General Details

Approved names: Teniposide, VM26, PTG, Thenylidene-Ligan-P.

Proprietary name: Vumon.

Manufacturer of supplier: Bristol-Myers Co. Ltd. & E R Squibb & Son

Presentation and formulation details: 5 ml ampoules containing a solution of teniposide 10 mg/ml. Each 5 ml also contains benzyl alcohol 150 mg, N,N-dimethylacetamide 300 mg, polyoxyetholated castor oil 2.5 g, absolute alcohol 4.7 g and maleic acid to adjust pH.

Storage and shelf-life of unopened containers: Ampoules should be protected from light and stored at room temperature. They are labelled with an expiry date.

2 Chemistry

Type: Podophyllotoxin derivative.

Molecular structure: Epipodophyllotoxin, 4-demethyl-,9-(4,6-o-2-thenylidene-beta-D-glucopyranoside).

Molecular weight: 656.

3 Stability Profile

Teniposide exhibits physical instability in aqueous solutions in varying periods of time depending on concentration, solution, and container type. The manufacturer recommends the following utility times for dilutions of the drug stored at either 4 or 25°C.

Infusion solution	Container type	Teniposide concentration (μg/ml)	Use within
0.9% sodium chloride	Glass	100	24 hr
	Glass	400	24 hr
	Plastic	100	8 hr
5% glucose	Glass	100	24 hr
	Glass	200	24 hr
Water for injections	Glass	100	24 hr
	Glass	200	24 hr
	Plastic	100	8 hr

Dilutions of teniposide at concentrations above 100 μg/ml in 0.9% sodium chloride and water for injection in plastic containers exhibit poor physical stability. At 100 μg/ml in 5% glucose in plastic containers, precipitation occurs within 4 hours at 25°C.

Precipitation occurs frequently in both glass and plastic containers at concentrations greater than those indicated in the table above. Discard solutions that show evidence of a precipitate.

Upon dilution, a slight opalescence may appear due to the surfactant present in the formulation.

Compatibility: 5% glucose and 0.9% sodium chloride.

4 Clinical Use

Main indications: Treatment of acute leukaemia.

5 Preparation of injection

Dilution: Dilute with the appropriate volume of infusion fluid. Refer to protocol.

Administration: Slow IV infusion.

Gloves for handling: Thick latex recommended.

Extravasation: Vesicant. Avoid extravasation. No specific management recommended.

6 Destruction of Drug or Contaminated Articles

Incineration: No specific information available.

Chemical: No specific information available.

Contact with skin: No specific information available.

7 UK Centres with a Known Interest in this Drug

None presently known.

8 Source of Information

1. NCI investigational drug data, 1989.
2. Bristol-Myers Co. Ltd. & E R Squibb & Son.

Prepared by T.Root

Glossary of Drug Names and Synonyms

Amsacrine	(BAN, USAN, pINN); AMSA; m-AMSA; Acridinyl; Anisidide. *Amsidine (Fr., UK); Amecrin (Denm., Norw., Swed.) Amsa (Canad.); Amsidyl (Austral., Ger.)*
Asparaginase	(USAN), COLASPASE (BAN), Crisantaspase, Erwinia L-aspariginase, L-Asparaginase, L-Asparagine Amidohydrolase. *Erwinase (UK), Crasnitin (Denm., Ger., Ital., Norw., UK); Crasnitine (Belg., Switz.); Elspar (USA); Kidrolase (Canad., Fr.); Laspar (S.Afr.); Leucogen (Spain); Leunase (Austral.)*
Azacytidine	Azacitidine (USAN, rINN); 5-Azacytidine; Ladakamycin. *Mysolar (USA)*
Bleomycin	Bleomycin Sulphate (BANM, pINNM) Bleomycin Sulfate (USAN). *Blenoxane (Austral., Canad., S.Afr., USA); Bleo Oil (Jpn); Bleo-S (Jpn); Blocamicina (Arg.); Verbublen (Canad.)*
Carboplatin	(BAN, USAN, rINN); JM8. *Paraplatin (Canad., UK); Paraplatine (Switz.)*
Carmustine	(BAN, USAN, rINN); BCNU *BiCNU (Canad., Fr., UK, USA); Becenun (Denm., Norw., Swed.,); Carmubris (Ger.); Nitrumon (Ital.)*
Cisplatin	(BAN, USAN, rINN); Cisplatinum, *cis*-DDP; CDDP; Cis-platinum; DDP; Peyrone's Salt. *Cisplatyl (Fr., Swed.); Citoplatino (Ital.); Neoplatin (Spain, UK); Placis (Spain); Platamine (S.Afr.); Platiblastin (Ger.); Platinex (Ger., Ital., UK); Platinol (Austral., Belg., Canad., Denm., Lux., Norw., S.Afr., Swed., Switz., USA); Platistil (Spain); Platistin (Denm., Norw., Swed.) Platosin (UK)*
Cyclophosphamide	(BAN, USAN, rINN); Cyclophospham. *Endoxana (UK); Carloxan (Denm.); Cycloblastin (Austral.); Cyclostin (Ger.); Cyclostine (Switz.); Cytoxan (Canad., USA); Endoxan (Austral., Fr., Ger., Ital., Neth., S.Afr., Switz.); Enduxan (Braz.); Genoxal (Spain); Neosar (USA); Procytox (Canad.); Sendoxan (Denm., Norw., Swed.)*
Cytarabine	(BAN, USAN, rINN); Arabinosylcytosine; Ara-C; Cytosine Arabinoside. *Alexan (Belg., Ger., Ital., Neth., Spain, Switz., UK); Arabitin (Jpn); Aracytin (Arg., Ital.); Cytosar (Austral., Belg., Canad., Denm., Jpn, Neth., Norw., S.Afr., Swed., Switz., UK, USA); Erpalfa (Ital.); Iretin (Jpn) Udicil (Ger.)*
Dacarbazine	(BAN, USAN, rINN); DIC; DTIC; Imidazole Carboxamide. *DTIC-Dome (Austral., Canad., Ital., Neth., NZ, S.Afr., Spain, Swed., Switz., UK, USA); Deticene (Fr., Ger., Ital., Neth., Switz.)*
Dactinomycin	(USAN, rINN); Actinomycin D (BAN); Meractinomycin. *Cosmegen, Lyovac (UK)*
Daunorubicin	Daunomycin Hydrochloride (BANM, USAN, rINNM); Rubidomycin Hydrochloride. *Cerubidin (Austral., Denm., Norw., S.Afr., Swed., UK); Cerubidine (Belg., Canad., Fr., Neth., Switz., USA); Daunoblastina (Ital., Spain)*
Doxorubicin	Doxorubicin Hydrochloride (BANM, USAN, rINNM); Adriamycin Hydrochloride. *Adriamycin (Austral., Canad.,*

	Norw., Swed., UK, USA); Adriblastin (Ger.); Adriblastina (Arg., Belg., Ital., Neth., S.Afr.); Adriblastine (Fr., Switz.); Farmiblastina (Spain)
Epirubicin	Epirubicin Hydrochloride (BANM, USAN, rINNM); 4'-Epiadriamycin Hydrochloride; 4'-Epidoxorubicin Hydrochloride; Pidorubicin Hydrochloride. *Farmarubicine (Fr.); Farmorubicin (Denm., Ger., S.Afr.); Farmorubicina (Ital., Spain); Farmoribicine (Fr., Switz.); Pharmorubicin (Austral., Canad., UK)*
Ethoglucid	(BAN); Etoglucid (rINN). *Epodyl (Austral., Neth., S.Afr., UK)*
Etoposide	(BAN, USAN, rINN); EPEG; VP-16; VP-16-213. *Etopol (Jug.); Vepesid (Austral., Canad., Denm., Ger., Ital., Norw., S. Afr., Spain., Swed., Switz., UK, USA)*
Fluorouracil	(BAN, USAN, rINN); 5-Fluorouracil; 5-FU. *Adrucil (Canad., USA); Arumel (Jpn); Carzonal (Jpn); Fluoroplex (Austral., Canad., USA); Fluorouracil (Austral., Belg., Denm., Neth., Norw., S.Afr., Swed., Switz., UK); Fluoro-Uracile (Fr.); Fluroblastin (Ger., S.Afr.); Fluoroblastine (Switz.); Timazin (Jpn); ULUP (Jpn)*
Idarubicin	(BAN, rINN); 4-demethoxydaunorubicin, Idarubicin hydrochloride (USAN).
Ifosfamide	(BAN, USAN, rINN); Iphosphamide; Isophosphamide. *Holoxan (Fr., Ger., Ital., Neth., Switz.); Mitoxana (UK); Tronoxal (Spain)*
Melphalan	(BAN, USAN, rINN); PAM; Phenylalanine Nitrogen Mustard. *Alkeran (Austral., Belg., Canad., Denm., Fr., Ger., Ital., Neth., Norw., S.Afr., Swed., Switz., UK, USA); Alkerana (Arg.)*
Mesna	(BAN, rINN); Mesnum. *Ausobronc Mesna (Ital.); Mistabron (Belg., Neth., S.Afr., Switz.); Mistabronco (Ger.); Mucofluid (Belg., Fr., Ger., Ital., Spain); Mucolene (Ital.); Sinomist (S.Afr.); Uromitexan (Fr., Ger., Ital., Spain, Switz., UK)*
Methotrexate	(BAN, USAN, rINN); Amethopterin; Methotrexatum; MTX. *Emtexate (Ger., Switz., UK); Emthexat (Norw., Swed.); Emthexate (Neth.); Farmitrexat (Ger.); Farmotrex (Denm.); Folex (USA); Ledertrexate (Belg., Fr., Neth.); Maxtrex (UK); Methotrexat (Ger.); Metotrexato (Arg.); Metrexan (Denm.); Mexate (USA); Tremetex (Swed.)*
Mithramycin	Plicamycin (BAN, USAN, rINN); Aureolic Acid. *Mithracin (Austral., Norw., UK, USA); Mithracine (Fr., Switz.)*
Mitomycin	(BAN, USAN, rINN); Mitomycin C; Mitomycine C. *Ametycine (Fr.); Mitomycin-C (Austral., S.Afr.); Mitomycin-C Kyowa (UK); Mitomycine (Belg.); Mutamycin (Canad., Norw., Swed., Switz., USA)*
Mitozantrone	Mitozantrone Hydrochloride (BANM); DHAD; Dihydroxyanthracenedione Dihydrochloride; Mitoxantrone Hydrochloride (USAN, rINNM). *Novantron (Ger., Switz.); Novantrone (Austral., Canad., Fr., S.Afr., UK)*
Mustine	Mustine Hydrochloride (BANM); Chlorethazine Hydrochloride; Chlormethine Hydrochloride (rINNM); HN2(mustine); Mechlorethamine Hydrochloride (USAN); Nitrogen Mustard. *Caryolysine (Fr.); Cloramin (Ital.); Erasol (Denm.); Mustargen (Canad., Switz., USA)*
Thiotepa	(BAN, USAN, rINN); TESPA; Thiophosphamide; Triethylene Thiophosphormide; TSPA. *Ledertepa (Belg., Neth.); Onco tepa (Spain); Tifosyl (Norw., Swed.)*

Vinblastine	Vinblastine Sulphate (BANM, rINNM); Vinblastine Sulfate (USAN); Vincaleucoblastine Sulphate; Vincaleukoblastine Sulphate; VLB (vinblastine). *Velban (USA); Velbe (Arg., Austral., Belg., Canad., Denm., Fr., Ger., Ital., Neth., Norw., S.Afr., Swed., Switz., UK)*
Vincristine	Vincristine Sulphate (BANM, rINNM); 22-Oxovincaleukoblastine Sulphate; Leurocristine Sulphate; Vincristine Sulfate (USAN). *Kyocristine (Jpn); Oncovin (Arg., Austral., Belg., Canad., Denm., Fr., Neth., Norw., Swed., Switz., UK, USA); Pericristine (S.Afr.); Vincasar (USA); Vincrisul (Spain)*
Vindesine	Vindesine Sulphate (BANM, rINNM); Desacetyl Vinblastine Amide Sulfate; Vindesine Sulfate (USAN). *Eldisine (Austral., Canad., Fr., Ger., Ital., S.Afr., Swed., Switz., UK); Enison (Spain)*

ABBREVIATIONS USED IN THIS GLOSSARY

Arg.	Argentina
Aust.	Austria
Austral.	Australia
BAN	British Approved Name
BANM	British Approved Name Modified
Belg.	Belgium
Braz.	Brazil
Canad.	Canada
Denm.	Denmark
Fr.	France
Ger.	West Germany
INN	International Nonproprietary Name
Ital.	Italy
Jpn	Japan
Jug.	Yugoslavia
Lux.	Luxembourg
Neth.	The Netherlands
Norw.	Norway
NZ	New Zealand
pINN	Proposed International Nonproprietary Name
pINNM	Proposed International Nonproprietary Name Modified
rINN	Recommended International Nonproprietary Name
rINNM	Recommended International Nonproprietary Name Modified
S.Afr.	South Africa
Swed.	Sweden
Switz.	Switzerland
UK	United Kingdom
USA	United States of America
USAN	United States Adopted Name